need to know

D1192572

First Aid

In association with the
Royal College of General Practitioners

Sheena Meredith MB BS MRCS (Eng) LRCP (Lond)
Consultant: Dr Vincent Forte BA MB BS MRCGP MSc DA

Collins

First published in 2006 by Collins
an imprint of
HarperCollins Publishers
77-85 Fulham Palace Road
London W6 8JB

www.collins.co.uk

Text and images:
© Book Creation Ltd, 2006
Back cover images:
Top and middle © Getty
All others © Alamy

A catalogue record for this book is available
from the British Library

ISBN-10: 0-00-721493-6
ISBN-13: 978-0-00-721493-8

Colour reproduction by Colourscan, Singapore
Printed and bound by Printing Express Ltd, Hong Kong

Contents

Foreword

In my role as Vice-Chairman of the Patient Partnership Group, people often tell me just how important it is for them to have easy-to-understand health information. This is never more true than when it comes to dealing with accidents and emergencies. Whether your situation calls for a doctor's attention, or you need an ambulance urgently, there are often many things that you can do to at the scene of the accident to improve the situation.

Written by a family doctor, *Need to know? First Aid* covers all the situations you might encounter and helps you to take effective action. You don't need to be trained in first aid to use this book, although I hope that it might encourage you to find out more, and perhaps take a course.

It has been endorsed by the Royal College of General Practitioners, so the information here combines a common sense approach with a large number of practical techniques. Most accidents happen in or around the home. Did you know, for example, that using the stairs is, minute for minute, one of the most dangerous things we do every day? You will find information on how to prevent accidents occurring, as well as being prepared for them by knowing what to keep in your first aid kit, for example.

There is a crucial section on life saving, which explains resuscitation techniques in children and adults. I would recommend that you give this a quick read-through before you put the book somewhere close at hand. This will ensure that you know what's covered and how to find the relevant information quickly should an emergency arise. You will see that there is a clear and logical A-Z listing of specific situations – from fainting and fever to splinters and sunburn. This will help you to deal with problems and emergencies without panicking, even if you have no first aid training.

On a practical note, keep your book in an easy-to-find place – and make sure everyone in the household knows where it's kept. Should you find yourself in an emergency, remember that you can quickly pull out the essential life-saving techniques information from inside the front cover.

Dr Catti Moss MA FRCGP
Medical Vice-Chairman, Patient Partnership Group
Royal College of General Practitioners

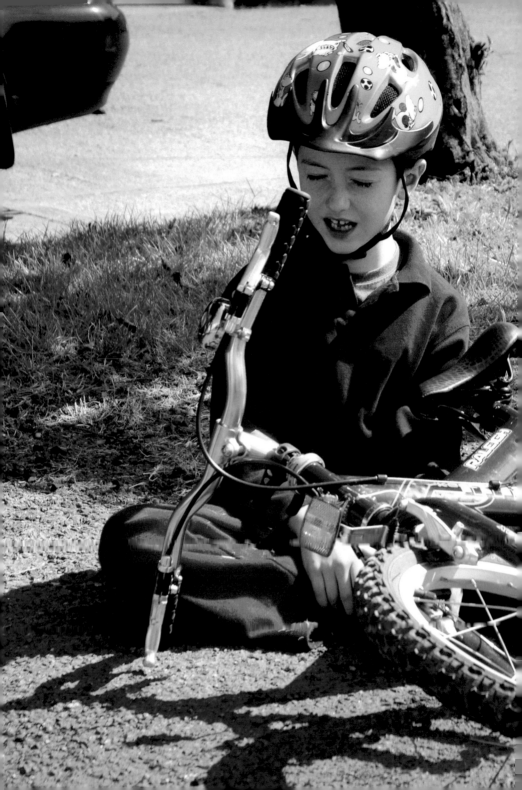

1 Be prepared

Having the essential items to hand can make all the difference when it comes to performing first aid. This section looks at common accident situations and also details the items you should keep to hand both at home and while out and about. The most important of these is a properly stocked first aid kit, which, alongside your own ability to keep calm and assess the situation at hand, will stand you in good stead for any incident that may arise.

Emergency priorities

Accidents and medical emergencies happen every day, any time, anywhere. Even if you have no first aid training, your intervention could help to limit the damage – and maybe even save a life.

Priorities in an emergency

Anyone could come across the scene of an accident, or suddenly be faced with an emergency at home. The key is to call for help, keep calm, assess the situation and know what to do in those vital minutes while awaiting help.

1 Stop to assess the situation – watch out for danger.
Your first aim is to avoid anyone else being put at risk –
for example, from oncoming traffic in a road accident.

2 Make sure it is safe to approach the scene
Never put yourself at risk – it is no help if you become a second casualty.
If you cannot help without endangering yourself or others,
call or send for help and keep others away.

3 Make the area safe
Do what you can to protect bystanders and others
from danger and protect the casualty from further danger.

4 Assess the victim
Check the casualty's response and condition (see pages 32–33).

5 Call for help

6 Resuscitate and treat injuries as necessary

Vital contact numbers

In an emergency there are several ways to summon help and assistance. In the majority of cases this will be by dialling 999 from any phone.

Emergency contact numbers:

Police, fire and ambulance services	**999**
European Union Emergency number	**112**
HMS Coastguard	**999**
Mine, mountain and cave rescue	**999**

Medical advice:

NHS Direct	**0845 46 47**
NHS24 (Scotland)	**08454 24 24 24**
Doctor	....
Local hospital	....
Dentist	....

Local utilities:

Gas supplier	....
Electricity supplier	....
Water supplier	....
Local council	....

First aid kits

A well-stocked first aid kit can make dealing
with minor accidents and injuries much easier.

Home first aid kit

As well as the full range of items that you will
wish to keep in the house, it's a good idea to keep
a first aid kit and other useful items in the car, in
case you encounter an emergency situation while
out and about. You can buy ready-made kits from
most pharmacies, or you can put together your own.
Store items in a clean, waterproof container with a
well-fitting lid, and clearly mark it 'first aid'.

Car first aid kit

As well as the essential items for a standard first aid
kit, you may also wish to carry:
- face shield or mask to protect you when
  performing resuscitation
- cardboard tie-on labels to identify casualties in
  major incidents
- notebook and pen for recording observations
- blanket
- cushions
- strong torch
- whistle
- survival bags – or rolls of kitchen foil –
  for keeping casualties warm and dry

must know

- Keep your first aid kit
  well stocked at all times
  or you may find it when it
  might be useful.

- Make sure everyone in
  the household or workplace
  knows where the first aid kit
  is kept.

Maintaining a first aid kit

1 If you use an item, be sure to replace it as soon as possible.
2 Check the contents regularly – at least once a year – and replace any out-of-date items.
3 Store in a high cupboard out of reach of small children.
4 Make sure the kit remains clean and dry: don't store it anywhere that could get damp, such as in a cupboard above the kettle or next to a window that's prone to condensation, or too hot, such as in a cupboard over the oven.
5 Make sure the kit is clearly labelled so anyone can locate it in an emergency.

other items to include

▶ bandage clips or safety pins
▶ disposable gloves
▶ tubular bandages for finger injuries
▶ large cotton-wool strips for padding
▶ eye pad
▶ thermometer
▶ wound-closure strips ('steri-strips')

The following items should be part of a standard first aid kit:

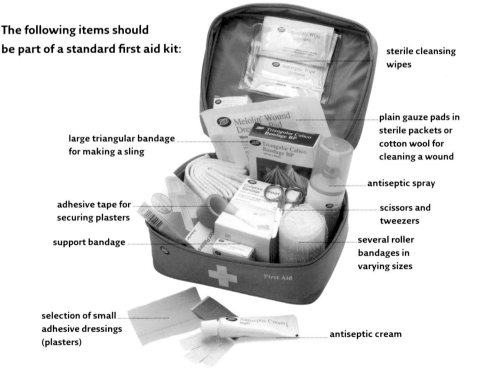

sterile cleansing wipes

plain gauze pads in sterile packets or cotton wool for cleaning a wound

large triangular bandage for making a sling

antiseptic spray

adhesive tape for securing plasters

scissors and tweezers

support bandage

several roller bandages in varying sizes

selection of small adhesive dressings (plasters)

antiseptic cream

Holiday first aid kit

It is well worth taking a comprehensive first aid kit with you when travelling, especially if you are going to remote areas, taking small children along or planning to engage in outdoor or sporting activities.

Travel first aid kit

You can buy a first aid kit specially for travel, or you can make up your own. Remember to include sufficient items for the size of your group and length of your trip.

As well as the dressings and other basic items listed in the standard first aid kit (see page 11), it may be helpful to take:

- first aid book or leaflet
- thermometer
- wound-closure strips ('steri-strips') or plasters
- vinegar – for jellyfish stings (small plastic catering sachets are ideal)
- rehydrating solution – for food poisoning and traveller's diarrhoea
- medicine spoon or medicine syringe (to measure fluids) – if travelling with babies or small children
- sunburn-relief spray or cream
- insect-bite/sting-relief ointment
- eye-flushing solution or sterile water
- chemical ice-pack
- chemical hot-pack

must know

In addition to your travel first aid kit make sure that you have the correct immunisations for your destination(s). Check with your doctor about what you might need and leave plenty of time as immunisations must be administered over several weeks.

Additional items that may be useful:

- sunscreen
- insect repellent
- water-sterilising tablets
- torch
- string or dental floss
  (very strong – has multiple uses)

Medicines for minor ailments

As finding a doctor in a foreign country can
be difficult – and may involve a language barrier
– it is a good idea when travelling to take a few
basic medicines to deal with minor conditions.
These include:

- mild painkillers – paracetamol,
  aspirin, ibuprofen
- anti-inflammatory and anti-fever medicine –
  aspirin, ibuprofen
- antihistamine cream – for insect bites
  and minor allergies
- anti-diarrhoea medication
- decongestant spray
- cough and cold remedies

Sterile supplies

In some parts of the world
it is advisable to take sterile
supplies for use by local medical
personnel in case you are in
an accident. These include:

- syringes and needles
- drip needle
- sterile suture kit

watch out!

- Never give aspirin
  to a child under 16.
- Always label medicines
  and keep a copy of the
  prescription for any
  prescribed medications.
- Do not pack scissors, needles
  or sharp implements in hand
  luggage – but don't send vital
  medicines through the hold.
- Remember that in some
  countries certain medicines
  may be illegal, for example
  codeine (present in some
  painkillers and anti-diarrhoea
  medicines).

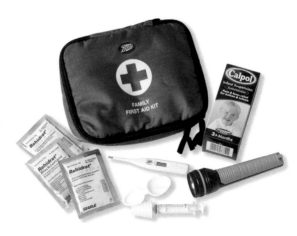

Common situations: accidents

Accidental injuries can happen anywhere – you never know when your first aid skills may be called upon. It's helpful to have read your first aid manual, so you know what to do if you are suddenly confronted by an unexpected event or incident and have to treat a casualty.

Where accidents happen

The vast majority of accidents happen at home, indoors. In the UK there are more than two million such incidents requiring medical attention each year. Roads and parking areas are the next most dangerous places, with more than 600,000 accidents per year. Next are accidents in the garden and other areas outdoors at home. So while you may feel safest at home, in fact this is the place you need to take most care.

Both children (see pages 18–19) and elderly people are at higher risk of accidents than adults of working age. Children, especially young children, are still developing their ability to move and co-ordinate and so are more likely to have purely physical mishaps. They are also less aware of danger and less able to protect themselves against hazards.

Older people are more frail, so are more likely to sustain injury even in minor incidents. They are also much more likely to be injured in falls (see page 17) – a major cause of accidents and, sometimes, with long-term complications.

must know

Who gets hurt?
Men outnumber women in the accident statistics – around six men are injured for every five women – and the male risk is even higher for fatal accidents. Men may engage in more risky activities – or they may take more risks in everyday life.

When are you most likely to get hurt?

Sporting activities are spectacularly dangerous, heading the league table of home and leisure injuries each year, and way ahead of the next most dangerous pastime – travelling. However, transport accidents are most likely to kill you, especially if you are male. Every year, more than 2,000 men, but fewer than 1,000 women, are killed while travelling. Falls are the next most common cause of death, affecting men and women almost equally, followed by poisoning – which is nearly twice as common among men. Other causes of accidental death, such as drowning or fire deaths, are far less common.

must know

There is a great deal you can do to help to prevent accidents occurring in the first place (see pages 168-183). If an accident does occur, a little first aid knowledge may enable you to treat minor injuries safely, know when and how to call for help (see pages 30-31), and stabilise the situation until the emergency services arrive.

Children are very accident prone, partly because their physical coordination is not fully developed, but also because their lack of experience - of accidents in particular - can make them overconfident.

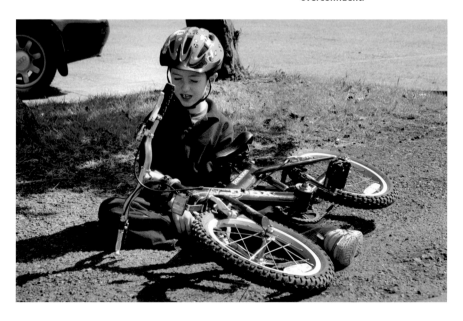

Common situations: accidents in the home

Home is not necessarily the safest place to be – indeed, it's where most accidents occur. More than 4,000 people die every year following household accidents. Most home accidents occur indoors – more than 2 million incidents per year, compared with more than half a million accidents in the garden and elsewhere outdoors around our homes.

Where danger lurks in the home

Surprisingly perhaps, the kitchen is only the second most dangerous area in our homes – although it's responsible for over a quarter of a million accidents per year. More than 30,000 of these involve knives, far exceeding accidents due to cookers and hobs: food preparation is more dangerous than cooking.

At the top of the danger list is our living space – living rooms, dining rooms, playrooms and studies. These are the scene of more than 300,000 accidents a year, perhaps because that's where we spend most of our waking time.

Also surprising is that the third most dangerous place to be is the bedroom, where more than 230,000 accidents occur annually. This makes it a slightly riskier place than the stairs, where more than 225,000 of us manage to hurt ourselves each year. However, as we spend relatively little time climbing or descending stairs, this is one of the most dangerous activities we undertake minute for minute.

did you know?

Every year, around 2.7 million of us are injured in accidents at home sufficiently seriously to seek medical treatment. This is on top of 1.6 million workplace injuries. Everyday life is hazardous.

Who gets hurt?

Children and elderly people are at the highest risk of domestic accidents. Almost everything in the home represents a potential hazard for a young child, from furniture and electric sockets to baths and household chemicals. Tripping and falling accidents are extremely common among young children, both because they are just learning to walk and haven't yet developed a full sense of balance, and because they are excitable and likely to move rapidly and with less awareness of their surroundings than adults. Also, many objects designed for adults – like chairs or coffee tables – are at just the wrong height for an active toddler. It's well worth spending some time child-proofing your home properly (see page 176-179) to avoid distressing trips to casualty.

Older people are similarly at high risk of falls: general ageing, various diseases and certain medications can all affect the sense of balance. Falls tend to be more serious in the elderly as they are generally less robust and more prone to break bones. So, again, it's important to look out for obvious hazards and guard against them where possible (see page 173).

A loose stair carpet or an item placed on one of the steps could lead to a fall.

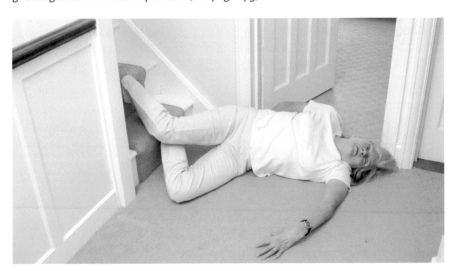

Common situations: accidents and children

Accidents are the leading cause of death in childhood in the UK – far more common than any childhood disease. An accident can occur in seconds, yet have lifelong or even life-threatening consequences.

Accidents and children

It's worth knowing, then, that many accidents could be prevented (see pages 168–183) – it is vital for parents and other carers to be alert to the dangers and do what they can to minimise them.

Road accidents in childhood

Road accidents are by far the most common cause of accidents in childhood. More than 5,000 children are killed or seriously injured each year on British roads - as passengers, pedestrians or cyclists. A child under 15 is more likely to die in a road accident than from any other cause. By the age of 16, one in 15 children will have been involved in a road accident. Many of these accidents are preventable (see page 180).

Children at home

Children are also at risk at home – more than half of all domestic accidents involve children under five. Special hazards for small children include:

- ► **drowning** - a child can drown in less than 5cm (2 inches) of water: baths, baby baths, sinks, lavatory bowls, paddling pools, garden ponds or water features and standing water in ditches and trenches are all a hazard
- ► **scalds** (see page 21)

did you know?

Baby product dangers
The number of accidents in 2002 due to cots or cradles was 3,957; in the same year 3,403 accidents were caused by high chairs; 2,317 by baby walkers; and 1,476 by baby bouncers. Even bottles and dummies have their risks with bottles scoring 1,251 and dummies 779.

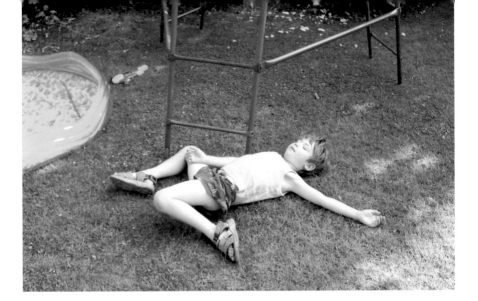

- **suffocation** – until babies can raise their heads, they are at risk from pillows, duvets, blankets and even soft toys
- **cot death** – this may be linked with infections, suffocation or overheating; the risk is reduced if babies are laid on their backs to sleep
- **choking** – children have very small windpipes where tiny objects may lodge and obstruct breathing
- **strangulation** – a child may become tangled in cords or ribbons, or get his or her head wedged in a small space or between bars
- **poisoning** – any household substance that is not intended to be swallowed poses a risk
- **injuries** - children often attempt to grasp attractive objects that are out of reach. Heavy furniture, such as a floorstanding bookshelf, may topple onto a child if he or she pulls it or tries to climb it. Explorations near a fireplace or heater can result in severe burns, and pulling on a table cloth can cause sharp or heavy tableware to fall on top of a child

Falls from trees, climbing frames and trampolines are common causes of injury in children.

did you know?

Balloon danger
As well as food and small objects like coins or beads, burst balloons are also a choking hazard for babies and young children.

Common situations: fire, burns and scalds

Around 100,000 people a year in the UK seek hospital attention for scalds or burn injuries, from fires or flames. Another quarter of a million people seek help from their GP for these injuries.

Fire, burns and scalds

Nearly 45 per cent of burns victims are children under five years old. Some injuries are trivial. Others can lead to permanent scarring, require years of intensive and often painful treatment; and some burns are fatal. On average, four people a week die from injuries caused by burns or scalds. Many of these injuries are preventable (see pages 174-175). Prompt first aid treatment - flushing with cold water for at least 10 minutes (see page 83) - can prevent scarring and long-term damage.

Fire!

Most deaths caused by fires are due to fires that start in the home. Half of all house fires start in the kitchen. Smoking materials and fires in electrical appliances are the next most common causes. A few basic safety precautions (see pages 174-175) could prevent many of these fires.

The main cause of kitchen fires is misuse of equipment and appliances, and the second most common cause is chip-pan fires. Most kitchen fires start between 10pm and 4am - people are more careless when they are tired or have been drinking.

Electrical fires can be caused by faulty or old appliances, or overloaded sockets.

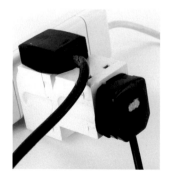

Some types of accident tend to be especially serious – clothing catching fire is likely to cause severe burns. It is worth knowing what to do (Stop, Drop, Wrap, Roll - see page 85), as well as taking sensible precautions with trailing or flammable clothing, long hair and tripping hazards near gas jets and open fires.

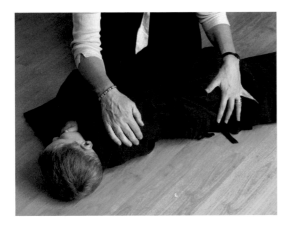

The 'Stop, Drop, Wrap, Roll' sequence will help smother flames. See page 85 for further information.

did you know?

Scalds
▶ Children have thin delicate skin, so they burn easily and quickly at lower temperatures than adults. They may be severely scalded if they play with the hot tap, or fall into a hot bath.
▶ About 450 children under five are admitted to hospital each year in the UK with severe scalds caused by hot bath water - the most common cause of scalding.
▶ More than 20 of these children die. Most survivors need prolonged and painful skin grafts and may be permanently scarred.
▶ Another 2,000 children have less severe injuries.
▶ Elderly people also have thin skin. Around 20 are killed each year by hot bath water.
▶ Water can still cause a nasty scald even 15 minutes after boiling.

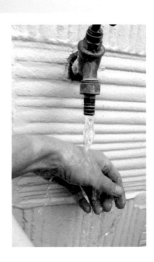

Common situations: accidents out and about

Travelling is one of the most dangerous activities we undertake. On average 107 people are killed or seriously injured each day on Britain's roads. The highest number of accidents occurs among pedestrians, followed by cyclists and then car occupants.

did you know?

Biker danger
Based purely on distance covered, a pedestrian or pedal cyclist is up to 16 times more likely to be killed than a car occupant – and a motorcyclist is at almost double that risk.

Hazards on the road

The statistics are hugely affected by how often each mode of transport is used. Mile for mile travelled, motorcycling is by far the most dangerous form of transport.

Children and elderly pedestrians are at the greatest risk of death or serious injury, and the majority of these accidents happen because the pedestrian crosses the road heedless of traffic, or masked from view behind a parked vehicle.

Safe driving, watching your speed, and basic road safety precautions could avoid tragedies.

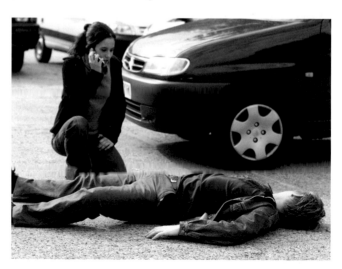

Calling for help is the first step to take at the scene of an accident.

Water

Activities in or near water are dangerous, even for adults. More than 400 people die in drowning accidents each year in the UK, and more than 20,000 people are injured while participating in water sports.

In the UK, water around the coast or in inland rivers, streams and ponds is sufficiently cold enough – even in summer – to cause hypothermia. This may make it impossible even for competent swimmers to get out of difficulty.

Children are at particular risk of drowning (see pages 178–179), particularly when unsupervised and away from home where more precautions may be taken – about 80 per cent of children who drown in ponds or home swimming pools are visiting relatives, friends or neighbours at the time.

Leisure time

Time spent enjoying leisure activities out and about can be hazardous. Sporting injuries are very common, especially among rugby players. Cricket, too, can cause nasty head injuries. Even an apparently sedate activity such as fishing has its dangers – carbon rods conduct electricity; hooks are sharp – causing more than 5,000 accidents requiring hospital attention each year.

Other types of accident are relatively modern. Bouncy castles now cause around 10,000 injuries per year – some involving permanent paralysis. This equipment should always be properly supervised and only people of roughly similar weights allowed on a bouncy castle together.

Another area of danger for children is the playground – more than 180,000 accidents occur in public, school or nursery playgrounds every year, with around three-quarters of these involving falls.

did you know?

Falls
- 40 per cent of all accidents requiring hospital treatment are due to falls
- 400,000 elderly people attend hospital each year after a fall
- falls are the most common cause of injury deaths in people over 75
- between one-third and a half of all over-65s sustain at least one fall in a year
- up to 140,000 people – mostly elderly die each year as a result of a fractured hip following a fall (see page 173)

Common situations: accidents in the garden

Accidents in the garden and outside the home account for over half a million injuries every year, of which more than 70,000 are due to gardening and over 18,000 involve children's play equipment.

Dangers outside the home

Another potentially dangerous activity is house maintenance – especially if the task involves ladders or power tools. People often get hurt tripping and falling over trailing hosepipes, loose paving slabs, slippery paths or uneven ground. Children are at particular risk of drowning in ponds, swimming pools, paddling pools or even rainwater butts (see pages 178–179). There are also bites and stings to contend with – only really dangerous if the victim is allergic to the venom – as well as possible plant allergies and children accidentally swallowing poisonous garden chemicals (see pages 146–148).

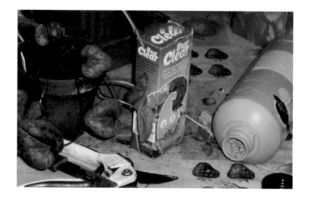

Do not leave garden poisons such as slug pellets in children's reach. Lock the blades of secateurs and keep all tools and toxic substances on a high shelf.

Lawnmower dangers

Lawnmowers cause more than 5,000 serious injuries a year, so it makes sense to treat them with respect and observe safety rules (see page 183). Injuries include:

- ▶ hand and foot injuries from lawnmower blades
- ▶ eye and other injuries from flying stone or gravel chips
- ▶ electric shock from slicing through a mower cable
- ▶ burns from refuelling a petrol mower while it is hot

Other garden hazards

Many accidents outdoors result from carelessness. It may be the stuff of comedy, but it is not funny to tread on the prongs of an abandoned rake and have the handle hit you in the face. This particular accident was responsible for more than 500 injuries requiring a visit to casualty in one year. Other common emergencies are caused by:

- ▶ animal bites
- ▶ poisoning from garden plants or berries
- ▶ burns from barbecues and bonfires

Do you need a tetanus jab?

By the time they reach their teens, most people have had five tetanus jabs and therefore have lifelong immunity. After a cut, a booster dose may be advised if the person is not sure if he or she has had five doses. If the wound is very tetanus-prone, contaminated with manure, say – then tetanus antibodies may be given.

---

did you know?

Trampoline injuries

Trampolines have become very fashionable and there has been a corresponding increase in trampoline injuries – around 50 per cent in five years. Much of this rise is the result of the popularity of large home trampolines. Here are some vital statistics:

- ▶ home trampolines cause more than 4,000 injuries to children a year
- ▶ children under six are especially vulnerable
- ▶ about 75 per cent of trampoline injuries occur when two or more people are using the trampoline at the same time
- ▶ where two people are together on a trampoline, the one who weighs the least is five times more likely to be injured
- ▶ more than half of all trampoline injuries occur despite adult supervision

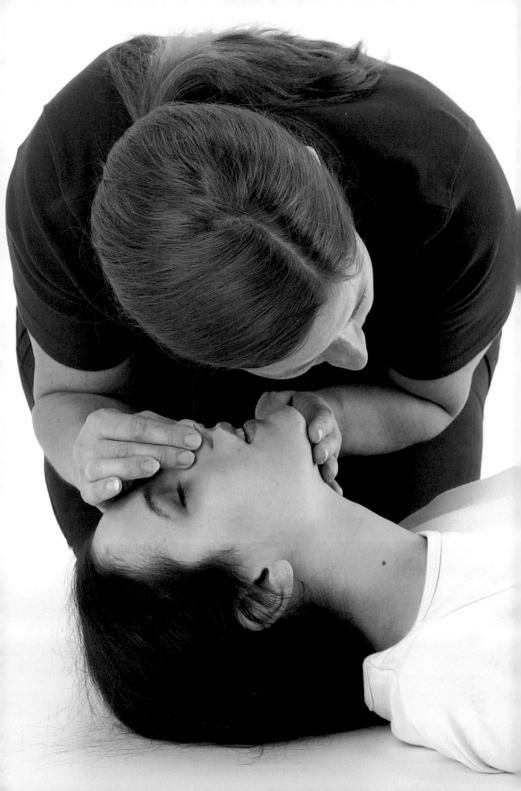

2 Life saving and first aid techniques

Being able to deal with a life-threatening situation promptly and effectively is a priceless skill. When someone's life is in danger, the first aider needs to stay calm, assess the situation and act – or not – in the most appropriate fashion. Life saving can be dangerous, dirty and unpleasant but it can also be relatively simple. These pages will help you to assess a situation, explain exactly what information you need to give to the emergency services as well as providing useful techniques about treating a casualty at the scene.

Emergency priorities

If you're going to help in an emergency, it's important first to consider your own safety – it's no good running to help a road accident victim and getting knocked down yourself.

In any emergency, it's important to keep calm and avoid panic responses. Before you rush in, stop, take a deep breath, and survey the scene carefully and logically. Don't try to deal with a situation in which you could be out of your depth – call or send for help.

Priorities in an emergency

1 Stop to assess the situation – watch out for danger. Your first aim is to avoid anyone else being put at risk – for example, from oncoming traffic in a road accident.

2 Make sure it is safe to approach the scene. Never put yourself at risk – it is of no help if you become a second casualty. If you cannot help a casualty without endangering yourself or others, call or send for help and keep others away.

3 Make the area safe. Do what you can to protect bystanders and others from danger. Protect the casualty from further danger.

4 Assess the victim. Check the casualty's response and condition (see pages 32–33).

5 Call for help.

6 Resuscitate and treat injuries as necessary.

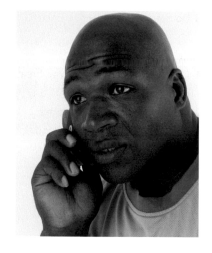

Assessing the situation

If you come across the scene of an accident, following some common sense rules can prevent further danger.

Be alert when approaching the scene
▶ Watch for fire, smoke, gas, leaking petrol or chemicals and electricity.
▶ If a vehicle involved is displaying a hazard-warning notice, such as 'toxic gas' or 'corrosive', do not approach. Call the police and describe the hazard by giving the information on the notice – there will be a letter or number code and a symbol.
▶ Do not allow bystanders to approach a hazardous area. For example, keep people at least 18 metres (60 feet) from a fallen power line (see page 109).

Safety in a road accident situation
1 Park behind the crashed vehicle(s) with your hazard lights on.
2 If possible, set up a warning triangle further back from the accident.
3 On minor roads, delegate bystanders to go back to warn oncoming traffic (make sure they walk facing the traffic).
4 Turn off the ignition and pull on the handbrake of all vehicles involved.
5 Do not allow anyone to smoke, in case of leaking petrol.

Assess the casualty
1 Check response, then airway, breathing and circulation (see pages 32-33). Deal with any immediate threats to life.
2 If there are multiple casualties, deal with life-threatening conditions first.
3 For more information on assessing casualties, see pages 44-47.
4 Call for help (see pages 30-31).

must know

Motorway hard shoulder hazard
The hard shoulder is not a safe place to be – many people get killed there while waiting for help to arrive. If a car breaks down on a motorway and has to pull over, the occupants must not stay in the car or stand on the hard shoulder. Instead, put on hazard lights, use a warning triangle if there is one, and then stand on the grass verge as far away from the hard shoulder as possible.

Getting help

One of the most important things you can do in any medical crisis or accident situation is to ensure that the emergency services are contacted fast, and to give relevant information as clearly and accurately as possible.

Call for help

If you can, send someone else to call for help so that you can stay with the casualty or remain at the scene to prevent further danger, and perhaps to give any immediately necessary treatment. Ask the person to come back to confirm that help is on its way.

If there is no one else around and you have to leave the scene, first take a moment to assess the situation and take any vital actions necessary (see pages 28-29).

How to contact the emergency services

In the UK, emergency calls are free from any telephone – whether at home, in a public call box or on a mobile phone. There are also emergency telephones situated at one-mile intervals along the sides of motorways – marker posts in between have arrows showing the direction of the nearest telephone

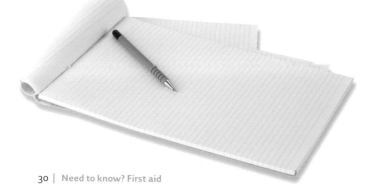

If you have to leave a casualty
1 Make the area safe.
2 Protect from further risks.
3 If necessary, move the casualty to a safer place.

Making an emergency call
When you make an emergency call, the operator will ask you which service you require. If anyone is hurt, ask for the ambulance service – they will inform the other services, such as the fire brigade, if necessary.

What information to give
Tell the operator:
1 Your name.
2 The precise location of the emergency – if possible the exact road name and nearest junction, with any noticeable nearby landmarks.
3 The nature of the emergency, such as a road accident or suspected heart attack.
4 How many people are affected, as well as their approximate age, sex and any other information you know about their condition, such as known allergies.
5 Whether there are any additional hazards, such as a suspected gas leak or icy roads.

watch out!

Do not hang up until told to do so by the operator.

ABC procedures

If you are confronted by a casualty or an accident, follow the 'DR ABC' checklist:

Danger   **Airway**
Response   **Breathing**
            Circulation

Danger
Assess the situation.
Is there any risk:
- to yourself?
- to bystanders?
- to the casualty?

YES

Do not place yourself in danger.
- Can you make the area safe?

NO

Call for help.

NO

YES

Check **Response**:
does the casualty respond to loud speech or a gentle shake or tap?
- *In a baby, gently flick the sole of the foot.*

YES

- Treat as necessary.
- Call for help if necessary.
- Monitor airway, breathing and circulation while waiting for help to arrive.

NO

Victim is unconscious.

Check **Airway**.

Check **Airway** (pages 34–35): does the casualty have a clear airway?	**NO**	▶ Call or shout for help. ▶ Clear the airway if possible (see page 34).

YES

Keep airway open (see pages 34–35).
Check **Breathing** (page 35).

YES

Check **Breathing** (page 35): is the casualty breathing?		Treat any life-threatening injury: ▶ Place in recovery position (see pages 42–43). *In a baby – hold in recovery position, which is in your arms with her head tilted downwards.* ▶ Call an **ambulance.** ▶ Monitor airway, breathing and circulation while waiting for help to arrive (see page 35).

NO

▶ Send someone to call an **ambulance**.
▶ *With a baby – take baby with you to call an ambulance.*
▶ Give two rescue breaths immediately (pages 36–37).

Check **Circulation** (see pages 38–39): is there a pulse?	**YES**	Continue with rescue breaths for one minute, then check **breathing** and pulse again (see page 35).

NO

▶ Ensure airway is still clear.
▶ Commence CPR (pages 38–41).
▶ Check breathing and circulation after one minute.
▶ Re-check every two minutes.

Still no breathing or circulation?
▶ Continue CPR until help arrives.
▶ Adult: 15 chest compressions: 2 rescue breaths.
▶ Baby/small child: 5 chest compressions: 1 rescue breath.

Breathing and circulation restored.

Airway and breathing

In an unconscious person, the tongue may fall backwards, blocking the airway and preventing effective breathing. Other obstructions may be present, for example, pieces of food, or foreign objects such as a coin or a marble in a child. Before taking any other action, it is vital to ensure that the airway is open and clear for breathing.

Opening the airway

Action

1 If possible, kneel beside the casualty.
   Place one hand on the person's forehead and gently tilt the head back.
2 If there is any obvious obstruction in the mouth, gently remove it.
3 Place two fingertips of the other hand underneath the point of the chin and gently lift it upwards to keep the airway open.
   In a baby – use one fingertip only under the point of the chin.

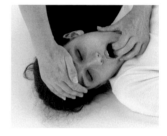

Gently remove any obstruction from the casualty's mouth.

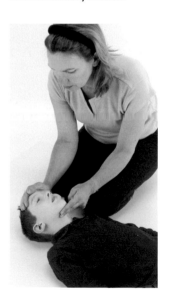

watch out!

▶ Do not try to clear the mouth by sweeping with your fingers
▶ If there may be an injury to the neck or spine, do not tilt the head back first. Handle the head very gently and use the jaw-thrust method (pages 152–154) to open the airway

Checking breathing

Action

1 Keep your hands in place to keep the airway open.
2 Kneeling over the casualty, place your face near the mouth. Listen for breath sounds and feel for exhalation against your cheek.
3 At the same time, look along the casualty's chest to see if it is rising and falling with breathing. Do this for up to ten seconds.

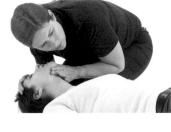

If the casualty is breathing:

1 Check for any potentially life-threatening injury (such as severe bleeding) and treat appropriately.
2 Place the casualty in the recovery position (see pages 42–43).
   In a baby – hold the baby in your arms, on his or her front, with the head down until help arrives. This will make sure the baby does not inhale vomit or choke on his or her tongue.
3 Call an ambulance.
4 Stay with the casualty until the ambulance arrives, continuing to monitor the airway, breathing and circulation. Be prepared to start resuscitation (see pages 38-39) if necessary.

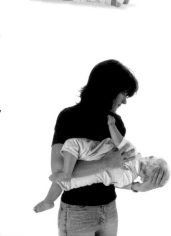

If you cannot detect breathing:

1 Send someone to call for an ambulance.
   In a baby – take the baby with you to call an ambulance.
2 Give two short rescue breaths immediately (see pages 36-37).
3 Proceed to resuscitation (pages 38-41).

This recovery position helps to stop a baby from choking on vomit or her own tongue.

Rescue breathing (mouth-to-mouth)

Without being able to take in oxygen from the air, a casualty who is not breathing may suffer serious brain damage or die. People can only live without oxygen for a few minutes.

By giving rescue breaths – what used to be called 'mouth-to-mouth' respiration or 'the kiss of life' – you can get enough oxygen into a casualty's lungs to keep him or her alive (your exhaled breath contains enough oxygen to do this). Rescue breaths may be enough to start the casualty breathing on his or her own. If not, you will need to combine breathing with chest compressions (see pages 38-39) to keep the person alive until the emergency services arrive.

Place your fingers under the casualty's chin and continue to pinch the nose as you take a breath.

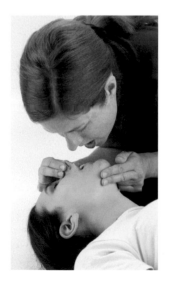

Adult and child (over 12 months old)
Action
1 Make sure the airway is still open (see pages 34-35).
2 Keeping the fingers of one hand steady under the chin, gently pinch the soft part of the casualty's nose between thumb and forefinger of your other hand, so no air can escape. Open the casualty's mouth with the hand that is under the chin.
3 Take a deep breath, then seal your lips around the casualty's open mouth, making sure that the join is airtight.
4 Blow steadily into the casualty's mouth, watching to see that the chest rises.

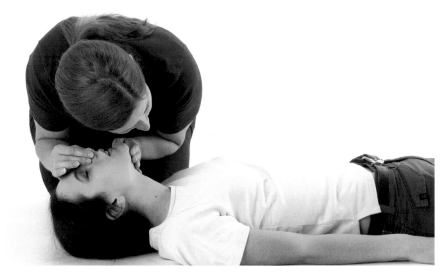

5 After about two seconds, take your mouth
away and watch the chest fall (see photo, above).
Keep pinching the nose.

6 After two good breaths, check for signs
of circulation (see pages 38-39).

Baby (under 12 months old)

Action

1 Make sure the airway is still open (see 34-35).

2 Keep the baby's head back with one hand on the
forehead and a finger under the chin.

3 Take a deep breath.

4 Seal your lips around the baby's *mouth and nose*,
making sure that the join is airtight.

5 Blow steadily until you see the baby's chest rise.

6 As soon as you see the chest rise, take your
mouth away and watch the chest fall.

7 Give two good breaths, and then check for
signs of circulation (see pages 38-39).

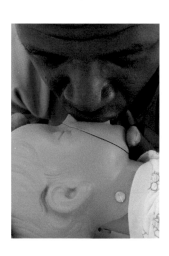

Cardiopulmonary resuscitation (CPR)

Most sudden deaths due to heart attacks occur outside hospital. If the heart stops, death can occur within minutes. Any serious injury, or incidents such as drowning or choking, may also stop the heart and lungs from functioning.

watch out!

Never use a real person for practising your CPR technique; you could cause injury.

The techniques of cardiopulmonary resuscitation (CPR) are used to keep someone alive until rescue services arrive, by manually pumping oxygen-containing blood to vital organs. CPR requires effective mouth-to-mouth breathing (see pages 36-37) to get oxygen into the lungs, plus chest compressions – pressing down on the breastbone – to squeeze blood out of the heart to the body, mimicking the action of normal contraction (heartbeat).

Checking circulation

This check should be performed after you have given two effective rescue breaths (see pages 36-37). If you know how to find the pulse at the wrist, test it there. However, the pulse of the carotid artery in the neck is often easier to find when a casualty is unconscious.

must know

In a baby – use your index and middle fingers to feel for a pulse on the inside of the upper arm.

1 Find the Adam's apple in the casualty's neck – the lump at the front of the throat.

2 Place the thumb and fingers of one hand into the grooves on either side of the Adam's apple (as shown in the picture). You should feel for a pulse first on one side and then on the other. If you are unsure, test the position by feeling your own neck with your other hand.

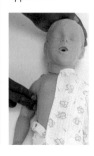

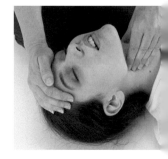

Pulse present:

1 Continue rescue breaths, re-check after one minute (the time it takes to give about ten breaths to an adult, 20 to a child under eight or a baby).

2 Call an ambulance if one is not already on its way.

No pulse:

Proceed immediately to chest compressions.

Action – cardiopulmonary resuscitation (CPR)

Before you begin, whatever the person's age, try, if possible, to lie the casualty on a firm surface – but **do not** attempt to move anyone with a possible neck or spinal injury. Kneel next to the casualty at about chest level.

CPR – adults

1 Using the first two fingers of one hand, locate the lower end of the rib cage. Then trace up to where the ribs meet the breastbone in the midline. Place one of your fingers over this junction, with your other finger just above it.

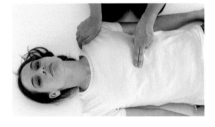

2 Place the heel of your other hand immediately above these two fingers.

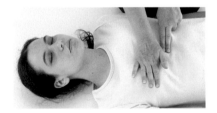

3 Now remove the finger markers and place the heel of this hand immediately on top of the other one. Interlock your fingers as shown, right.

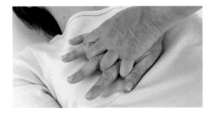

4 Holding your hands in this position, lean well forward over the chest, keeping your arms straight. Press firmly downwards on the breastbone, aiming to depress the chest by about one-third of its total depth.

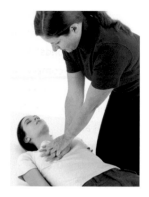

5 Allow your hands to come back up, maintaining the same hand position, so the chest wall springs back up too. Do 15 compressions, aiming for a rate of about 100 compressions per minute (a fast count – about five compressions in three seconds. It may help to count out loud). After 15 compressions, stop and give two rescue breaths.

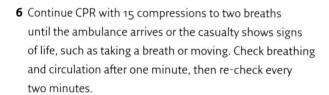

6 Continue CPR with 15 compressions to two breaths until the ambulance arrives or the casualty shows signs of life, such as taking a breath or moving. Check breathing and circulation after one minute, then re-check every two minutes.

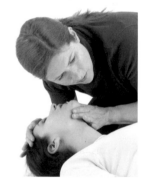

7 If the casualty's heart and breathing start again, place in the recovery position (pages 42–43). Make sure someone has called an ambulance and monitor the casualty until help arrives. Be prepared to start resuscitation again if necessary.

CPR – children under 8

1 Find the correct hand position on the breastbone as for an adult, but use the heel of one hand only to give compressions. Lift the fingers of this hand slightly, to avoid compressing the child's ribs.

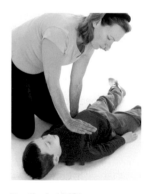

2 Lean over the child's chest, keeping your arms straight, and press firmly downwards on the breastbone, aiming to depress the chest by about one-third of its total depth.

3 Pull your hand up to allow chest wall to rise.

Use the heel of one hand only to give chest compressions to a child under the age of eight.

Repeat for five compressions, aiming for a rate of about 100 compressions per minute (five compressions in three seconds).

4 After five compressions, stop and give one rescue breath. Continue to alternate five compressions with one breath for one minute, then stop and call an ambulance if one is not already on its way.

5 Continue CPR at a rate of five compressions to one breath until the ambulance arrives or the child moves or takes a breath.

6 If the child's breathing and circulation are restored, place in the recovery position (see pages 42–43). Make sure someone has called an ambulance and monitor the child's condition until help arrives. Be prepared to start resuscitation again if necessary.

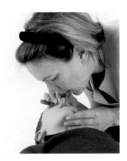

Give a child under eight one rescue breath for every five chest compressions.

CPR – babies up to 12 months

1 Imagine a line drawn between the baby's nipples.

2 Place the first two fingers of one of your hands a finger's width below this point on the midline.

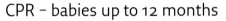

3 Using **just these two fingers**, press firmly down on the chest, aiming to depress the chest by about one-third of its total depth.

4 Lift your hand up to allow chest wall to rise.

5 Repeat for five compressions, aiming for a rate of about 100 compressions per minute (five compressions in three seconds).

6 After five compressions, stop and give one rescue breath. Continue to alternate 5 compressions with one breath.

7 Make sure someone has called an ambulance and continue CPR until help arrives.

Use two fingers on a baby when doing compressions.

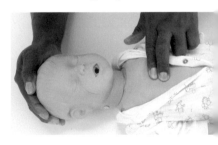

Give a baby one rescue breath after every five chest compressions.

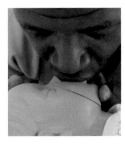

Recovery position

One of the biggest dangers for an unconscious person is suffocation. Placing an unconscious casualty in the recovery position may save his or her life.

The recovery position keeps the airway open, allows saliva or vomit to drain from the mouth, and is a stable position in which to leave a casualty if necessary.

watch out!

If you suspect a neck or spinal injury, and the casualty is unconscious, follow the procedures for spinal injury outlined on pages 152–154.

Action for adults and children

1 Kneel beside the casualty and remove glasses and any bulky objects in pockets.
2 Straighten the casualty's legs.
3 Place the nearest arm at right angles to the body, with the elbow bent up at a right angle and the palm upwards.

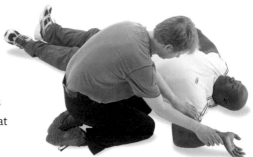

4 Take the casualty's far arm and bring it across the chest towards you, placing the back of the hand against the casualty's cheek.
5 Grasp the casualty's far-side leg and bring the knee upwards, keeping the foot on the floor. Pull on the raised knee to roll the casualty towards you.

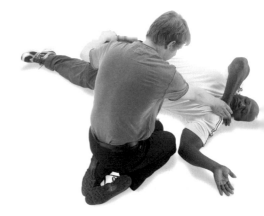

6 With the casualty on his side, tilt the head back to maintain an open airway. Prop the casualty's head on his hand if necessary to keep the head tilted and the airway open.

7 Adjust the uppermost leg so that the hip and knee are both bent at right angles.

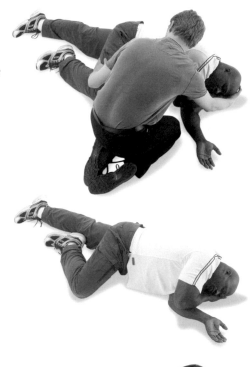

8 Monitor the casualty's condition until the ambulance arrives. Be prepared to start resuscitation if necessary (see pages 36–41). If you are still awaiting help after 30 minutes, reposition the casualty unless there are other injuries, such as broken bones. Roll him onto his back and put him in the recovery position from the other side.

---

must know

▸ If the casualty is already lying on his side, you do not need to roll him onto his back before putting him in the recovery position. Instead, ensure an open airway by tilting the head back and then adjust the limbs until they are in the recovery position.

▸ The recovery position should **only** be used if you are sure that an unconscious casualty is breathing and has an adequate circulation.

Action for a baby

1 Hold the baby in your arms with her head tilted downwards until help arrives. This will make sure she does not inhale vomit or choke on her tongue.

2 Check her breathing at regular intervals.

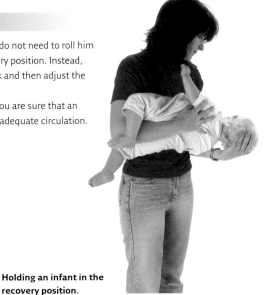

Holding an infant in the recovery position.

Assessing the victim

The first priority in any emergency is to ensure safety, and then to look for and treat any immediate threats to life. Keep calm, follow the DR ABC drill, call for help and give resuscitation if necessary (see pages 32–33).

First priorities:

Danger

Response

Airway

Breathing

Circulation

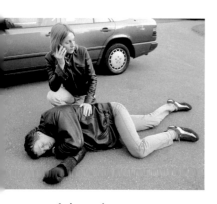

A clear and accurate assessment of the casualty and the surrounding area is vital when contacting the emergency services.

Next, look for and treat any major injuries or conditions that could become life-threatening, such as:

- ▶ severe wounds
- ▶ severe bleeding
- ▶ shock, or anaphylactic shock
- ▶ major burns or smoke inhalation
- ▶ major fractures (breaks in bones)
- ▶ internal injuries
- ▶ spinal (back or neck) injuries
- ▶ heart attack

If you suspect any of these conditions, call an ambulance at once, then begin appropriate treatment while awaiting help.

General principles

Whatever the circumstances, observe hygiene principles (see page 164).

1 Identify the condition(s).

2 Assess severity and the need for help.

3 Offer treatment as appropriate.

4 If out in the open, move to warm dry place if possible, or shelter casualty.

5 If possible, note the casualty's name and address (in case he or she loses consciousness).

6 Ask the casualty whether he or she would like you to contact a relative or friend.

7 Safeguard the casualty's possessions and send to hospital with the casualty.

Take a history

If casualty is conscious, ask about:

1 The history of the accident or incident – what happened, when it started, whether anything like this has happened before.

2 Symptoms – what the casualty feels, such as pain or numbness?

3 Movements – check that the casualty can move all limbs and digits (fingers and toes).

What to look for

Even if the type of injury appears to be obvious, be alert for other, hidden, injuries.

▶ Look for wounds, bleeding, deformity, skin discoloration or burns. Check for fluid or blood leaking from nose or ears.

▶ Listen to breathing – is it noisy, laboured, fast or slow?

▶ Look for clues from the scene – is there evidence of the cause of the accident, or of possible problems such as electric shock, hypothermia, drugs overdose or poisoning?

▶ Does the casualty have any medicines? These may give a clue to the problem; for example, angina medication suggests risk of heart attack.

watch out!

What not to do
▶ Never put yourself in danger.
▶ Don't move a casualty unless vital to remove from danger.
▶ Don't move a casualty's head or neck after a fall or an impact, this is unless necessary for resuscitation.
▶ Don't remove clothing unless necessary for assessment or treatment.
▶ Don't give anything to eat or drink: the casualty may need an anaesthetic.

Consider the casualty's age

Elderly casualties:

▶ may have existing illnesses such as heart disease

▶ are more likely to break bones in a fall

▶ are vulnerable to circulatory failure and shock

▶ are vulnerable to hypothermia

Babies and children:

▶ may need a modified form of resuscitation (see pages 40–41)

▶ are vulnerable to poisoning (see pages 146-148)

▶ are more at risk from burns (page 83)

Unconscious casualty

As well as the signs above, look for:

▶ MedicAlert bracelet – warns of serious medical conditions

▶ adrenaline auto-injector – possible anaphylaxis

▶ insulin for injection, glucose or sweets, or smell
of pear drops on the breath – the victim may be diabetic

▶ inhaler – may be asthmatic

▶ epileptic medication

▶ heart medication – possible heart attack

▶ any drugs or containers – poisoning or overdose

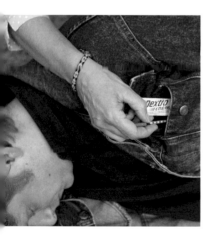

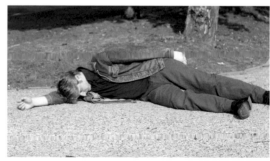

People can lose consciousness for various reasons. Sometimes, there may be clues in a pocket or among the person's belongings.

Incoherence or disturbed consciousness

Possible causes include:

- intoxication (page 136)
- overdose (page 145)
- diabetic incidents (page 98)
- head injury – concussion (page 124)
- post-epilepsy (page 116)
- heat stroke (page 128)
- hypothermia (page 133)

Dealing with multiple casualties

In a major incident such as a road accident, a train crash or even a terrorist attack, there will be multiple casualties and associated chaos and panic. Remain calm. Inform emergency services, direct bystanders to help or to leave the area, and give emergency aid until help arrives.

Priorities in any incident with more than one casualty

1 Call for help immediately (see pages 30–31).
2 Assess the scene (see page 29).
3 Make the area safe if possible (see page 29) – this may include alerting nearby residents or workplaces of any continuing danger.
4 Ask for help from bystanders.
5 Treat life-threatening injuries first.
6 Do not move a casualty who is seriously injured unless necessary for safety or effective treatment.
7 Ask minor casualties ('walking wounded') to wait away from the main accident scene.
8 Do not disturb anything at the scene unless necessary in order to get a casualty to safety – there may be evidence vital for later investigation of the incident.

must know

Triage
The process of deciding which casualties need most urgent attention is known as triage. As a general rule, an unconscious casualty is the most in need of help. If you think a casualty is dead, leave him or her, in order to help those who could be saved.

watch out!

The noisiest casualties are not necessarily the most severely injured.

Types of dressing

Any open wound – one where there is a break in the skin – should be covered with a dressing to help prevent infection until new skin has had a chance to form over the damaged area.

Adhesive dressings
Ordinary adhesive dressings ('plasters') suitable for small cuts and grazes come in a variety of sizes and shapes, including ones designed specially for fingers and heels. They can be made of waterproof plastic or fabric, and have a small area of gauze to cover the wound with a self-adhesive border all round. Plastic plasters should be used in all food preparation areas as fabric types are considered less hygienic. Fabric can also fray and may be less durable.

Some people are allergic to the fabric types, and a few to the adhesive used even on plastic ones – but you can buy hypoallergenic brands. Always check that the casualty is not allergic before you apply an adhesive dressing.

Gauze dressings
Larger wounds may require a gauze dressing, some of which have a thin plastic film on one side to stop the dressing sticking to the wound. Dressings are available in a variety of sizes. They are usually sold in individual sterile packets and may incorporate a dressing pad already attached to a roller bandage. Sterile eye pads are also available.

Bandages
There are three main types of bandage:
▶ roller bandages – the standard bandage strip
▶ triangular bandages – for large dressings, immobilisation when there is a suspected fracture, or to make a sling

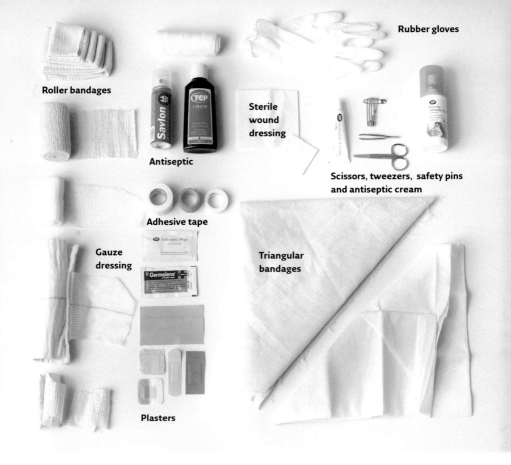

Rubber gloves

Roller bandages

Antiseptic

Sterile wound dressing

Scissors, tweezers, safety pins and antiseptic cream

Adhesive tape

Gauze dressing

Triangular bandages

Plasters

▶ tubular bandages – designed to fit on fingers and toes to secure dressings or support injured joints. Larger sizes are available to support ankle or knee joints

Bandages come in a variety of sizes and materials. Usually you need bandage clips, adhesive tape or safety pins to secure them in place, but self-adhesive bandages are available.

Other materials

To dress wounds you will also need:

▶ disposable latex gloves

▶ antiseptic lotion, spray or ointment, or sterile cleansing wipes

▶ plain gauze pads or cotton wool for cleaning a wound

▶ scissors and tweezers

Cold compress

Applying a cold compress to the area of an injury reduces bruising and swelling because blood vessels constrict when they are cold, reducing the blood's circulation.

A cold compress or ice pack also lessens pain in many conditions. This treatment is useful for everyday knocks, sprains or strains, as well as to reduce the pain of insect stings. A cold compress on the forehead may ease a fever or headache.

Making a cold compress
Soak a cloth – a tea towel or flannel is ideal – in cold water (preferably iced water) and wring it out. Apply to the affected area for as long as it helps, and renew as often as needed. You may need to refresh in chilled water every five minutes or so.

Making an ice pack
Place ice cubes or, better still, crushed ice in a strong plastic bag and wrap in a cloth, such as a tea towel. Alternatively, use a packet of frozen peas – you will not be able to eat them afterwards, but the pack is readily re-usable. You can also buy instant chemical cold packs.

watch out!
Do not leave an ice pack on for more than 10 minutes at a time as this may damage the tissues or impair circulation.

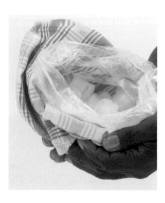

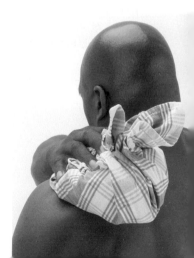

RICE technique

The RICE technique is the general treatment for sprains and strains, and may help with any knock or blow where bruising is a possibility.

RICE stands for:
Rest
Ice
Compression
Elevation

Resting the injured part of the body prevents further damage. It reduces blood flow to the area, and so the chance of swelling and bruising. An ice pack or cold compress (see opposite page) may help to relieve pain and also reduces blood flow to the injured area.

Compression of an injured limb, using a pressure bandage or similar, prevents leakage of blood and fluid into the tissues surrounding the injury – a common response to trauma – and so helps to reduce swelling and bruising. By elevating the affected part above the level of the heart, blood flow is reduced and this too reduces the risk of bruising.

These techniques together help to lessen any immediate pain and reduce the ongoing effects of a soft-tissue injury. If pain or other symptoms persist, seek medical attention.

watch out!

Allow a little movement from time to time, especially in lower limbs, to protect against DVT (deep vein thrombosis).

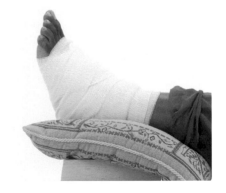

Bandaging

Bandages can be used to secure dressings, to apply pressure to control bleeding or reduce swelling, and to support or immobilise injured limbs.

Applying bandages – general guidelines

▶ Ensure that the site of the wound is clean before applying a dressing. Wash your hands and use disposable gloves whenever possible (see page 164).

▶ Before applying a bandage, have the casualty sit or lie down in a comfortable position, with the injured part supported.

▶ Offer reassurance if the casualty is upset or alarmed.

▶ Ensure privacy and calm if possible – ask people who are not helping to move away.

▶ Explain what you are going to do. If possible, get the casualty to help – by supporting the injured part, applying pressure or holding the end of a bandage. This may distract the casualty from pain or anxiety.

▶ Face the casualty if possible, standing or kneeling on the injured side.

▶ Leave fingers and toes exposed if possible, so that you can check circulation later (see page 54). Secure the bandage firmly but not too tightly.

▶ If using a bandage to hold a dressing in place, you only need to bandage sufficiently to keep the dressing secure. If using a bandage for support, extend it well beyond the area that is injured, if possible by an equal amount on each side.

▶ When bandaging around a joint, start from the inner side of the joint, using diagonal turns.

▶ Secure bandages in place with tape, safety pin or clip. If using a safety pin, always have the point facing downwards to minimise the risk of injury if it comes undone.

▶ If using knots to secure a large bandage or sling, use a reef knot. Position it away from the site of injury and away from any bony prominences, for comfort.

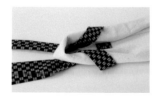

A reef knot is an effective way of securing a bandage.

Elbow or knee bandage

1 Start with the arm or leg bent, if possible.

2 Place the end of a roller bandage on the inside of the joint and wind it around the joint with a half-turn overlap, so it is secure.

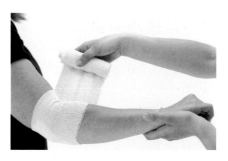

3 Make a turn of the bandage just above this. Overlap the first turn by about half its width, with the overlap starting on the inside of the joint.

4 Do the same with a turn just below the joint, starting on the inside and passing the bandage diagonally down, then making a turn below the joint that overlaps the lower edge of the first turn.

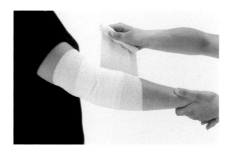

5 Continue to wind the bandage diagonally above and then below the joint, increasing the area covered by overlapping each time.

6 End with two straight turns and secure the bandage in place.

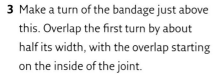

watch out!

Checking circulation

For limb injuries, check circulation regularly (see page 59) to ensure that the bandage is not too tight, and that any swelling is not constricting the limb under the bandage.

Hand or wrist bandage

1 Place the end of a roller bandage on the inner side of the wrist, by the base of the thumb.

2 Make two straight turns around the wrist.

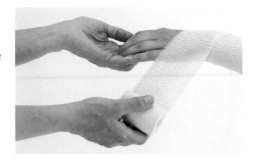

3 Pass the bandage diagonally from the inner side of the wrist across the back of the hand to the last joint of the little finger.

4 Pass the bandage straight across the palm side of the fingers to the last joint of the index finger.

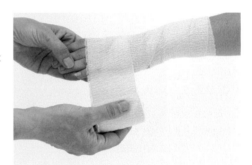

5 Pass the bandage diagonally across the back of the hand to the wrist.

6 Repeat these diagonal turns, overlapping the bandage each time until the hand is covered, leaving the thumb free.

7 End with two straight turns around the wrist and secure the bandage in place.

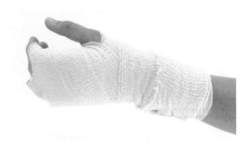

Foot bandage

Use the same technique as for a hand bandage, but begin at the base of the big toe and wind around the foot and ankle, leaving the heel uncovered.

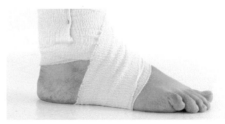

Arm sling

1 Ask the casualty to support the injured arm at the elbow, with the hand slightly above the horizontal.

2 Drape a triangular bandage under the arm, with its long side down the unaffected side of the body, the top round the neck and the point level with the elbow on the affected side.

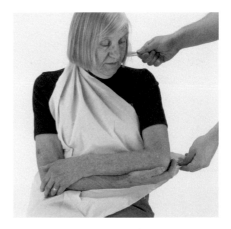

3 Fold the lower end of the bandage up over the forearm and tie it securely over the shoulder with the knot resting in the hollow above the collarbone.

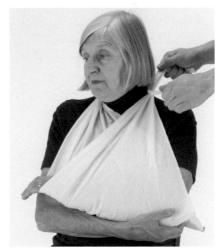

4 Fold the point of the bandage forwards over the elbow, tuck in and fasten with a safety pin.

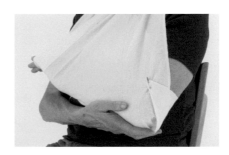

Elevation sling

1 Ask the casualty to support the injured arm at the elbow with the fingertips resting on the opposite shoulder.

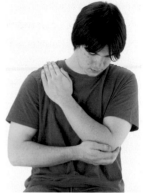

2 Drape a triangular bandage across the body and over the arm, with its long side down the unaffected side of the body, the top round the neck and the point level with the elbow on the affected side.

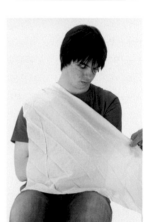

3 Ask the casualty to move the unaffected arm away and tuck the base of the bandage under the affected arm, with the top end wrapped around the hand.

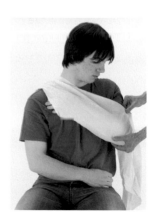

4 Take the lower end of the bandage up over the back and tie it securely over the shoulder with the knot resting in the hollow above the collarbone. Tuck in any loose fabric at the elbow and fasten with a safety pin.

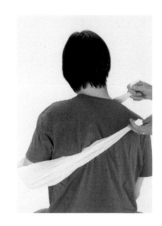

Head bandages

1 Fold a hem along the long edge of the bandage and place along the casualty's forehead, with the point hanging down the back.

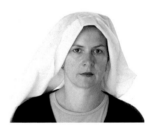

2 Cross over the two ends behind the point and in a knot at the front.

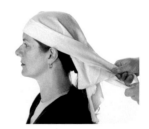

3 Pull the point down until the bandage cap is tight, then bring it up over the top of the head and secure with a pin, or tuck in over the crossed ends of bandage.

must know

Use a roller bandage to apply pressure to a bleeding scalp wound. Wind the bandage around the head as necessary on top of the pad or dressing. A triangular bandage can be used to hold a dressing in place.

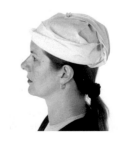

Improvising

When giving first aid, it helps a lot to have access to proper, sterile dressings and clean bandages. This is why it's always worth keeping a well-stocked first aid kit both at home and in the car (see pages 10-11). However, in an emergency you can often improvise with items that are to hand.

▶ Cling film makes an excellent burns dressing – discard two turns of the roll to ensure a clean surface to apply to the wound.

▶ Plastic bags are useful if you have no cling film, and make a convenient covering for wounded hands or feet. They are also helpful for making ice packs (see page 50) and for transporting things to hospital with the casualty, from a severed finger (page 167) to samples of pills.

▶ Any piece of clean material torn into strips will substitute for a roller bandage.

▶ A headscarf or large square of material folded diagonally will do instead of a triangular bandage.

▶ A button-up jacket can help to support an arm with minor injuries – insert the hand of the affected side through a convenient gap to rest it on the button below (a Nelson position).

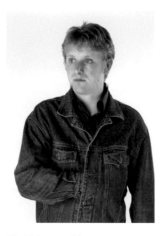 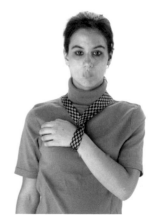

The Nelson position can support an arm with minor injuries.

A neck tie can make a simple but effective loop support.

- For a suspected fracture, a stronger support is obtained if you take the corner of the jacket and secure it with a safety pin to the collar or upper chest area on the affected side, with the arm resting in the fold created.
- A belt, tie or pair of tights can serve to support an injured arm. Place behind the neck and fasten at the front in a wide loop, then twist the front of the loop to form a second, smaller loop. Gently place the hand of the injured arm in the loop.

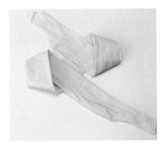

A belt, as well as a bandage can support an injured arm. Make two wide loops, as above.

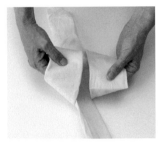

Bring the loops together and gently place the arm through the loops.

Signs that circulation may be impaired

- limb appears swollen
- blue skin, prominent veins
- numbness
- cold, pale skin with a waxy appearance
- tingling or pins and needles
- pain
- inability to move fingers or toes

Even without these signs, you should check the circulation once the bandage is in place and then every 10 minutes or so. Do this by pressing a nail or fingertip until it goes pale, then releasing and watching for the return of the normal pink colour. If this is slow or absent, the bandage may be too tight and you should loosen it until normal skin colour returns.

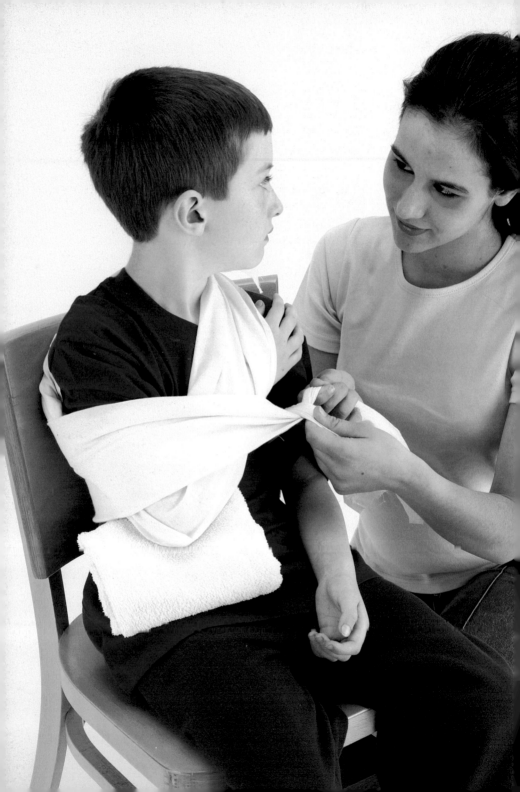

3 A–Z of first aid treatments

Together with the first aid knowledge you have gained in the first two parts of this book this section contains all the information you need to know about how to deal with any first aid situation. Entries are listed alphabetically for ease of use and cross referenced in the index as well as between the entries themselves.

In the event of an accident, keep calm, assess the situation, make the area safe and check the casualty. Always call for help immediately before beginning life saving treatment and attending to any injuries as necessary.

First Aid A-Z

Abdominal injury

Injuries to the abdomen – the region of the body between the chest and the hips – may arise from blows, crushing or penetration. There is a risk of damage to internal organs.

Signs of abdominal injury
- bruising or bleeding
- signs of shock (see pages 149-150)
- bleeding from the mouth or anus

Action
1. If you think that someone has an abdominal injury, call an ambulance at once.
2. Lie the casualty down and loosen belts and tight clothing.
3. Cover any obvious wound with a sterile dressing or clean pad.
4. Cover any protruding abdominal contents such as the intestines with cling film or a clean plastic bag. Apply a dressing on top, secured by a bandage if necessary.
5. If blood seeps through the dressing, apply a second dressing on top.
6. Monitor airway, breathing and circulation and be prepared to start resuscitation if necessary (pages 34-41).

Abdominal pain
If a person has severe abdominal pain without a history or signs of injury, call a doctor – he or she may have appendicitis or another serious condition.

watch out!

Abdominal contents could protrude through the wound if the victim vomits, coughs or sneezes. Apply gentle pressure on top of the dressing.

must know

Winding – pain, distress and difficulty breathing after a blow to the abdomen – usually eases within a few minutes. If not, there may be a more serious internal injury.

Allergy

An allergic reaction occurs when the body's immune system treats a normally harmless substance as if it were a foreign invader. Symptoms vary from person to person.

did you know?

Allergies affect around one in four people in the UK at some time in their lives.

watch out!

▶ Do not leave the person alone until the initial symptoms have started to improve – there is always a risk of a severe reaction developing.
▶ Dial 999 if symptoms worsen.

Causes

People can develop an allergy to anything. Common causes include drugs and medicines, foods, pollen and insect bites or stings. An asthma attack (see page 74) may be triggered by an allergic reaction. The most common foods that people suffer a reaction to are milk, eggs, peanuts, nuts, fish, shellfish, soya and wheat.

Typical allergy symptoms

▶ a red, blotchy, spreading skin rash
▶ raised bumps or weals, like nettle rash (hives, urticaria)
▶ blistering
▶ intense itching at the site of contact, or around the mouth for something eaten
▶ swelling of a body part
▶ puffy or watery eyes
▶ sneezing and a runny nose
▶ nausea or vomiting
▶ abdominal pain
▶ diarrhoea

A severe allergic reaction can trigger anaphylactic shock (see pages 66-67).

Action

1 Ask whether the victim has suffered an allergic reaction before.

2 If the victim is aware of a previous severe reaction, call an ambulance at once.

3 For mild symptoms antihistamine drugs may help, but always advise the person to seek medical advice.

4 If the person is having an asthma attack, help him to use his inhaler (see page 74).

5 Treat any vomiting or diarrhoea (see page 100).

6 Call an ambulance at once if any swelling develops around the face, especially the lips or tongue, or if the person is distressed or has any breathing difficulties.

7 Be prepared to provide emergency treatment if a severe allergic reaction (anaphylaxis) develops (see pages 66-67).

must know

The most common trigger for anaphylactic shock is an insect sting.

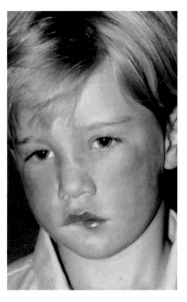

Hives are characterised by raised white or yellow lumps and an area of red inflammation.

want to know more?

For more information about allergies, contact Allergy UK. The charity runs a website (www.allergyuk.org) as well as a helpline (01322 619898, from 9am to 5pm, Monday to Friday).

Severe allergy

Allergies are becoming more and more common, and severe reactions are also increasing. Victims may go into anaphylactic shock, meaning that the reaction is affecting the whole body.

Anaphylactic shock involves a rapid, severe and sometimes life-threatening reaction to a trigger substance that an individual is allergic to, leading to a dramatic fall in blood pressure. This reaction is potentially life-threatening.

Almost anything can trigger such a reaction, and it may develop within seconds or minutes of contact with the trigger. Common causes are insect stings; things eaten, such as nuts or shellfish; and drugs and medicines. People who know they are severely allergic may carry emergency adrenaline for auto-injection to counter the allergic response – immediate treatment can be life-saving.

must know

Who is at risk?
The main causes known to trigger severe allergic reactions are peanuts, shellfish, wasp and bee stings, latex – such as in gloves, elastic and condoms – and drugs such as penicillin. Those especially at risk are people with a history of allergies, for example, asthma, hayfever or eczema.

Signs of severe allergic response

▶ rapidly spreading, red, raised skin rash (urticaria or hives)
▶ intense itching
▶ swelling of lips, tongue and throat, and sometimes hands and feet
▶ puffiness around the eyes
▶ breathing difficulties – coughing, wheezing, shortness of breath
▶ rapid pulse, extreme anxiety
▶ shock (see pages 149–150) and collapse

Action

1 Call an ambulance immediately and say the casualty may be in anaphylactic shock.
2 Check whether the victim carries an adrenaline auto-injection device and, if necessary, help him or her to use it.
3 Help the person to sit in a comfortable position that best aids breathing.
4 Treat for shock (see pages 149–150).
5 Be prepared to start resuscitation if necessary (pages 38–41).

Using an adrenaline auto-injector

1 The auto-injector will work even through clothing – do not waste time trying to undress the victim.
2 Remove the cap.
3 Hold the other end of the injection device against the victim's outer thigh, **at right angles to the skin**.
4 Press hard – the injection will be triggered automatically.
5 Hold the device in place for 10 seconds.
6 Remove the device and massage the site for a further 10 seconds.
7 Some fluid will remain in the syringe – this is normal.
8 Dispose of the device safely.

watch out!

Emergency adrenaline should be injected **only** into the outer thigh, not the buttock area.

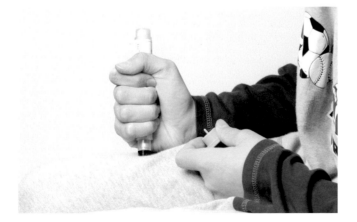

Always check to see if the casualty has left special instructions about how to use their medication.

Animal bites and scratches

With any type of bite or scratch, treatment centres on reducing the chances of infection. Insect bites are common and most cause only temporary and mild discomfort.

Animal bites – including those from humans which are increasingly common in cases of assault – are very likely to become infected because the mouth is full of germs. Scratches may also become infected, and those from cats in particular may cause a spreading infection called cat-scratch disease. Occasionally, people are bitten by snakes, though relatively few are venomous.

Signs of an animal bite
▶ puncture marks from teeth
▶ scratches
▶ pain, redness and swelling around the wound
▶ nausea, vomiting, sweating and disturbed vision from snake bites

Action
1 If someone has been bitten by a snake, call an ambulance.
2 Wash the area of the bite or scratch thoroughly with an antiseptic wash, or with soap and water.
3 Cover with a sterile dressing.
4 Always seek medical attention for an animal bite or deep scratch since a tetanus injection may be needed.

For a snake bite
While waiting for medical help to arrive, hold the affected part down below the level of the heart.

must know

Bites
Human bites must be treated with antibiotics if the skin is broken.

watch out!

Snake bites
▶ Snake venom is still toxic even when the snake is dead.
▶ If the snake has escaped, notify the police.

Ankle and foot injury

Sprained ankles are common, as are impact injuries to the feet. Such injuries are usually caused by jumping or falling from a height onto a hard surface.

A sprained ankle is usually due to a twisting or wrenching force when a person trips or loses their footing. It may be difficult to distinguish a sprain (see page 156) from a broken bone (fracture).

Signs of ankle or foot injury
▶ pain that's worse on movement or weight-bearing
▶ inability to stand or walk
▶ swelling, bruising or deformity

Action
1 If you suspect a fracture, seek urgent medical attention. Support the leg as with a leg injury (see pages 138-139).
2 For a sprain, use the RICE procedure – rest, ice, compression and elevation (see page 51).
3 Once the swelling has subsided, the ankle will still look very bruised. Protect and support it with with a bandage.

watch out!

There is a risk of permanent damage from an unattended fracture – treat all severe ankle injuries as fractures until shown otherwise.

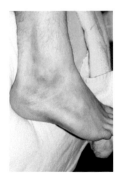 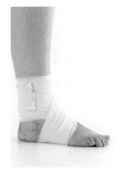

must know

Is it a sprain or a strain?
▶ A sprain involves damage to ligaments around a joint.
▶ A strain involves damage to the muscles.
▶ Both cause pain, swelling and muscle spasm, although a strain is usually less severe.

Arm injury

Fractures or dislocations of the arm are common injuries. They can affect the shoulder, upper arm, elbow, forearm or wrist.

Signs of arm injury
▶ pain, increased by movement of the injured area
▶ tenderness over site of injury
▶ swelling or deformity
▶ bruising

In an elbow injury:
▶ difficulty straightening arm
▶ tingling or numbness in fingers

In a forearm injury:
▶ an open wound, sometimes with bone ends protruding

The upper arm bone, called the humerus, is most often broken in a fall, and the typical victim is an elderly person. The humerus can also be fractured by a direct blow.

The forearm, the region between the elbow and the wrist, has two bones called the radius and ulna, which can be broken either by a direct blow or by a fall onto the outstretched hand. These injuries may be open fractures – where the bone ends protrude through the skin – because the bones have relatively little tissue surrounding them to cushion the impact.

The joints of the arm can also be injured. The shoulder may be dislocated by a pulling force, a fall directly onto the point of the shoulder, or a fall onto the

watch out!

Fractures may go undetected if the casualty does not experience much pain. It can also be difficult to distinguish a fracture from a dislocation. Therefore, treat any moderately severe injury as a fracture until proved otherwise. Always seek medical attention.

must know

Keep the casualty warm with blankets to decrease the possibility of shock (page 149).

outstretched hand. At the elbow, fractures or dislocations often occur after a fall onto an outstretched hand, especially in children. These injuries need careful handling as there is a risk of damage to blood vessels and nerves around the elbow from the broken bone ends.

The most common wrist injury is a fracture of the lower end of the radius, called a Colles' fracture. Falls onto the outstretched hand may also break one of the tiny carpal bones that make up the wrist itself. Because of the way the carpal bones are organised, wrist dislocation is rare – though sprains are common.

Action – shoulder and upper arm injury

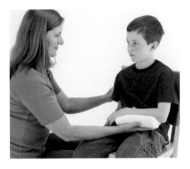

1 Ask the casualty to sit down. You will need to immobilise the arm and shoulder by placing the arm in a sling.

2 Place the arm in a comfortable position across the chest and ask the casualty to support it.

3 Use a triangular bandage as an arm sling (see page 55). Place soft padding – such as wads of cotton wool or a folded towel – between the injured arm and the bandage where it lies against the chest. Tie the sling in position to support the arm.

4 Tie a broad bandage over the sling and around the chest to secure the sling in place, avoiding the injured area if possible.

5 Take or send the casualty to hospital in a sitting position.

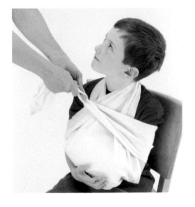

Action – elbow injury

If the elbow can bend, treat as an upper arm injury (see page 71). If the elbow cannot bend, do not attempt to move or bandage it.

1 Lie the casualty down and place soft padding between the elbow and the body to support the arm. Avoid touching the site of the injury.

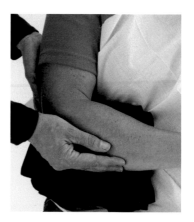

2 Call an ambulance.
3 While waiting, check the pulse by placing three fingers just below the victim's wrist crease on the thumb side. Tell the ambulance personnel if the pulse weakens or disappears.

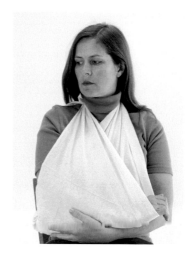

watch out!

▶ Never try to reposition a dislocated elbow or shoulder.
▶ Do not allow the casualty to eat or drink as he or she may need an anaesthetic.

Action – forearm injury

1 Ask the casualty to sit down.

2 Place the injured arm across the chest and ask the casualty to support it.

3 Treat any open wound (see page 164).

4 Place a rolled-up newspaper under the forearm as a splint and secure with bandages.

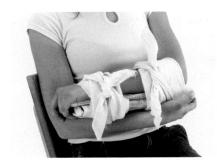

5 Place a triangular bandage ready for an arm sling (see page 55).

6 Place soft padding around the arm – use cotton wool, a rolled hand-towel or other material.

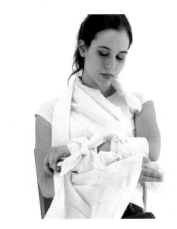

7 Tie the sling in position and support with a broad bandage on top, tied around the chest.

8 Take or send the casualty to hospital.

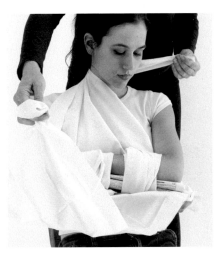

Asthma attack

In an asthma attack the air passages narrow, making it difficult to breathe. An attack can make a person feel like they are suffocating.

**Young children
often use a spacer
device to help
them take their
medication.**

Signs of an asthma attack

► a feeling of tightness in the chest
► difficulty breathing or speaking
► wheezing when breathing out
► grey skin and blue lips
► coughing, especially during attacks at night

Action

1 Help the person into a comfortable position – sitting up and leaning slightly forwards is often helpful.
2 If the person has a reliever inhaler (blue cap), help him to find and use it.
3 Encourage the person to breathe slowly.
4 Use a second inhaler dose if necessary after three minutes.
5 Be prepared to start resuscitation (see page 36) if necessary.

Call an ambulance if:

► this is the first attack
► a second dose of inhaler has no effect
► breathing is getting progressively more difficult

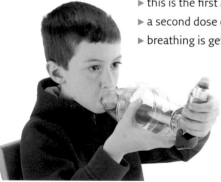

Back pain

Lower back pain is extremely common, usually due to a minor injury to the back muscles after heavy lifting or sudden twisting of the spine.

Back pain can also arise when one of the soft discs separating the spinal bones (vertebrae) becomes damaged, or moves ('slipped disc'). Back pain should always be evaluated thoroughly by a doctor, especially if it follows any kind of trauma or accident, to exclude the possibility of neck or spinal injury (see pages 152-154).

Action

1 If there is a history of an accident, check for spinal injury (page 152).
2 Call an ambulance if there are signs of spinal injury or if back pain is accompanied by impaired consciousness, headache and fever, any loss of movement or sensation in the legs, or incontinence.
3 With spinal injury ruled out, help the casualty to lie in a comfortable position on a firm surface.
4 Offer mild painkillers.
5 If rest and painkillers do not alleviate pain within 48 hours, call a doctor.

must know

What to look for:
▶ pain, usually in the lower back, often increased by movement
▶ pain radiating down the back of one leg
▶ tingling or pins and needles in the toes
▶ spasm of the back muscles, so the back is held stiffly

watch out!

Do not ignore any unusual symptoms – seek urgent medical advice.

Bites and stings

Insect bites and stings are common and usually not serious, but they may provoke severe allergic reactions. For animal bites, see page 68.

Symptoms of a bite or sting
- ► sudden sharp pain – the victim usually knows he has been stung or bitten
- ► localised redness, soreness and swelling in the region of the sting or bite

Action

1 Call an ambulance if the person is allergic to stings or if signs of anaphylaxis develop (see pages 66-67).

2 If the casualty has been stung in the mouth, give cold water or ice cubes to suck, and take or send to hospital at once – there is a risk of swelling of the airway.

3 If the sting is still present, remove it by scraping with a credit card, your fingernail or other flat surface.

4 Use an ice pack to reduce pain and swelling.

5 Pour vinegar on jellyfish stings to reduce pain.

6 Call an ambulance for any form of marine sting or wound.

did you know?

When treating a jellyfish sting, urine is a useful substitute for vinegar to reduce pain.

watch out!

Never remove a sting with tweezers - this will simply squeeze more poison into the wound.

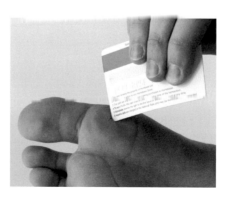

A sting can be removed by scraping it with a credit card.

Black eye

A black eye is often the result of a blow to the eye or bridge of the nose. It is a type of bruise in which burst blood vessels leak under the skin.

Symptoms of a black eye
- swelling around the eye
- dramatic bruising spreading out around the eye socket
- pain

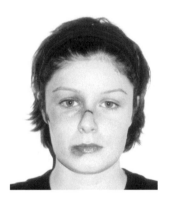

Anyone with a black eye should have it checked by a doctor to confirm the absence of any serious injury.

Action
1 Encourage the victim to lie down and rest, to reduce blood flow to the area.
2 Apply a cold compress such as a flannel soaked in cold water or a pack of frozen peas wrapped in a towel.
3 Use the compress for 10 minutes as soon as possible after the injury. Reapply after 20 minutes if necessary.
4 See a doctor urgently if there is any disturbance in vision.
5 Seek urgent attention if there is clear or blood-stained fluid leaking from the nose or ear.

Bleeding

Bleeding may occur with any wound that causes a break in the skin, and heavy bleeding can be alarming. You can help in an emergency by remaining calm and knowing how to respond.

Other types of bleeding can also occur. A closed wound may cause bruising – bleeding under the skin – such as in a black eye (page 77). Usually the bruise will heal on its own. However, bruising may be a sign of more serious internal injury.

Bleeding can also occur from orifices, such as a nosebleed (page 144), or vaginal bleeding following childbirth (page 88) or miscarriage (page 142).

Any bleeding or leakage of clear fluid from the nose or ears following a head injury (see page 125) is a possible sign of skull fracture and needs urgent medical attention.

Signs to look for
- an obvious wound with external bleeding
- bruising and other signs of injury such as broken bones
- shock, if the casualty loses a lot of blood (see pages 149–150)
- signs of internal bleeding after a trauma – pain, pattern bruising (the imprint of an object), confusion, deteriorating consciousness

watch out!
- Seek urgent medical attention for severe bleeding, shock, major wounds, embedded objects, broken bones or if you suspect internal bleeding.
- Internal bleeding into the skull, abdomen or chest can occur after trauma and may be difficult to detect.

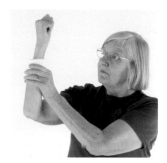

Keeping an injured limb above the level of the heart will reduce the circulation to the part and staunch the flow of blood.

Action

Your aim is to stem any serious bleeding. Provided there is no embedded object in the wound (if there is, see page 166), follow these steps:

1 Put on disposable gloves if available.
2 Use a dressing pad or your hand to press firmly
   directly over the wound – ideally, get the casualty to do this.
3 Raise an injured limb above the level of
   the heart to help staunch the flow.
4 Lie the casualty down if possible, with the legs slightly raised.
5 When blood flow lessens, secure a dressing
   over the area with a moderately tight bandage.
6 If the wound continues to bleed,
   place a second dressing over the first one.
7 Call an ambulance.
8 While waiting for help, monitor the casualty's condition,
   and be prepared to start resuscitation if necessary (see pages 38–41).
   Check that the bandage is not interfering with circulation (see page 59)
9 Assess for and treat shock (page 149) or broken bones (see pages 44-47).
10 Treat open wounds, ensuring good hygiene
   to avoid infection (see page 164–167).

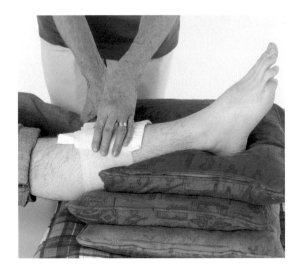

Secure a moderately
tight bandage when
the blood flow
lessens.

Blisters

A blister is a local swelling on the skin containing fluid. It is usually painful if touched.

Blisters may result from friction, burns, infections, chemicals or allergies. Typical causes of blisters include new shoes, sunburn and chickenpox. Most blisters heal by themselves without treatment.

Blister symptoms
- pain
- distinct, fluid-filled lumps under the skin
- clear fluid leaking from blister

Action
If a blister is in an area subject to friction – such as where a shoe rubs or a clothing strap chafes – or if one bursts spontaneously, cover with a sterile dry dressing. Otherwise leave well alone.

When to see a doctor
- Seek medical help if a blister becomes red, hot, swollen or filled with pus – this suggests an infection that may need treatment.
- Seek medical help for extensive blistering or blisters due to severe burns, shingles or eczema.

watch out!

It is best not to burst a blister – the skin over the top helps keep infection out until a new layer of skin forms underneath.

Boils

A boil is a collection of pus under the skin, due to an infection. Most boils form in infected hair follicles. The face, neck, armpits and groin are common sites.

Identifying boils

▶ pus-filled spot under the skin, usually coming to a distinct 'head'
▶ area is usually red, hot, swollen and painful

Action

1 Using a hot compress may help bring the boil to a head and speed healing. Hold a flannel soaked in hot (but not scalding) water on the area for 10 minutes at a time, several times a day.
2 If a boil bursts, clean the area with antiseptic and leave it open to the air to heal.

When to see a doctor

▶ Seek medical help if a boil gets very large or spreads – it may form a carbuncle (collection of boils) or an abscess (with pus tracking further inside the skin) and need treatment.
▶ Talk to your doctor if you suffer from recurrent boils – your doctor may wish to test for diabetes, as people with this condition are especially vulnerable to boils.

watch out!

Resist the urge to burst a boil – you could spread the infection.

Bumps and bruises

Any blow to the body may cause bruising, which is due to bleeding under the skin. Most bumps and bruises heal by themselves.

A bruise, as identified by a discoloration of the skin, may occur immediately after a blow to the body or hours or even days later. Sometimes a bump causes swelling – especially on the scalp, where there are many blood vessels, which can result in alarmingly large bulges. Most bumps and bruises are not serious, but it is important to be alert for signs of more serious injury, especially following a blow to the head (see page 124).

If someone is bruising very easily and often, they should see a doctor as this could be a sign of a blood disorder.

Action

1 Ask the casualty how the bump or bruise happened (if not obvious) as this can indicate the severity of the injury.
2 With a bump to the head, if you suspect that the casualty has lost consciousness at any time, seek medical help at once.
3 Raise the affected limb if possible and apply firm pressure.
4 Apply an ice pack (see page 50) for five to ten minutes to reduce pain and minimise swelling.
5 Treat any other injuries, such as sprains and strains (see pages 156–157).

want to know more?

If you or someone you know is or could be a victim of domestic violence, contact the National Domestic Violence Helpline on 0808 2000 247. The freephone line is staffed 24 hours a day. You can also visit www.womensaid.org.uk

Burns and scalds

Burns may be caused by flames, hot objects, scalding water or steam, chemicals, friction, electricity or radiation. They are categorised according to their depth.

As a rule, more severe burns involving deeper tissues are less painful, because nerve endings are destroyed. Loss of fluid is an immediate danger, and later there is a risk of infection.

Signs of a burn
- pain – although this may be absent in a severe burn
- red or black skin
- blistering and weeping of the skin
- swelling of the affected area

Action
1. Immediately flush the affected area with cold running water from a tap for at least 10 minutes. In an emergency any source of cold, non-flammable liquid (such as milk) will do.
2. Remove any rings, bracelets, watches, anklets or other items that could be constricting.
3. Remove clothing from the affected area – cut it away if necessary – but leave any parts that are stuck to the burn.
4. Cover the burn with cling film or a sterile, non-stick dressing (the type with a layer of clear plastic material next to the wound) – this helps prevent infection from sticking to the wound.
5. Monitor the victim while awaiting help and be prepared to treat signs of shock (see pages 149–150) or to start resuscitation (page 36–41) if necessary.

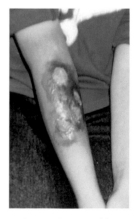

Make sure the wound is free from clothing but leave any that is stuck to the burn.

Call an ambulance

You should seek medical attention for all but the most trivial of burns, especially if:

▶ the victim is a young child
▶ the burn involves an area bigger than the size of the victim's hand
▶ the airway is affected
▶ the hands, feet, face or genitals are affected
▶ the burn goes around the entire circumference of a limb.

Chemical burns

1 Do not approach the area unless it is safe to do so.
2 Do not place yourself in danger.
3 Remember that some chemicals may burn through plastic or rubber gloves.
4 Call an ambulance.
5 Flood the burn with cold water for at least 20 minutes (longer than for a heat burn) and do not touch the victim until you are sure the chemical has been washed away. Then remove all clothing that may be contaminated.
6 Monitor the casualty and be prepared to treat shock (see pages 149–150) or to start resuscitation (pages 36–41).

watch out!

Look out for:
▶ signs of shock (see page 149)
▶ signs of smoke inhalation – high risk of breathing difficulties (see opposite)
▶ entry and exit burns from electricity – high risk of cardiac arrest (see pages 126-127)
▶ chemical contamination (see left)

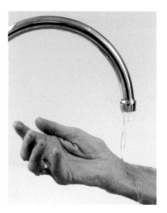

Flood the affected area under cold water.

watch out!

▶ Do not touch the burnt area directly, as this may introduce infection.
▶ Do not use any kind of fabric or fluffy material (such as cotton wool or gauze) on a burn – it could stick and be difficult to remove.
▶ Do not use any fat, oil, ointment or other greasy substance on a burn – it seals in heat and makes burns worse.
▶ Do not burst blisters – they protect delicate tissues beneath until new skin can form.

Burns caused by a fire

After any fire in a confined space, the casualty may have breathed dangerous smoke or hot gases into the airway. There may be:

▸ soot around the nose and mouth

▸ swelling of mouth and throat

▸ hoarse voice

▸ difficulty breathing

Call an ambulance at once and monitor the airway very closely. Give ice or sips of cool water to try to reduce swelling. Be prepared to start resuscitation at any time (see pages 36–41). Do not leave the casualty alone.

Smothering the flames

If a person or their clothing is on fire, follow this sequence:

Stop ▸ moving around only 'fans the flames'

Drop ▸ get the victim on the ground

Wrap ▸ if possible, wrap the victim in a rug, blanket or other heavy material

Roll ▸ roll the victim over on the ground. The flames should be extinguished.

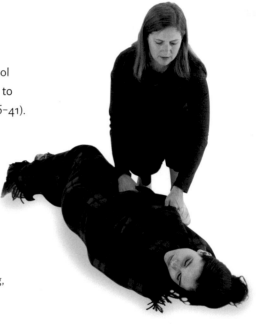

Chest injury

Chest injuries may be due to blunt trauma (such as a sudden blow or punch), crushing forces or penetrating wounds.

watch out!

If the casualty's chest has been crushed for longer than 15 minutes, do not attempt to remove the crushing object (see page 97).

The effects of a chest injury may include lung damage and broken ribs. Chest pain arising without an injury is extremely common, especially among older people.

Signs of chest injury include pain, which is worse on breathing; shallow, uneven or laboured breathing; a sucking noise on breathing in; coughing blood; bloodstained fluid seeping around the wound; and a crackly sensation when feeling around the wound (this is caused by air leakage). The victim's skin may look grey and the lips blue. He or she may well be experiencing a sense of panic.

Action

For a penetrating wound:

1 Lean the casualty towards the injured side.

2 Seek urgent medical attention – if there is a penetrating or crushing injury, call an ambulance. Be prepared to start resuscitation if necessary (pages 36-41).

3 Place a thick sterile dressing or clean pad over the wound.

4 Cover with an airtight material such as clingfilm or a clear plastic bag. Tape this firmly on three sides, leaving one side free – this allows air to escape but not enter.

For suspected rib fractures:

1 Support the arm on the affected side with a sling (see page 55) and lean the casualty towards that side.

2 Arrange transport to hospital.

must know

Place a breathing but unconscious casualty in the recovery position (page 42) with the injured side downwards – this enables the unaffected lung to work best.

Chest pain

Older people often experience chest pain, without injury. If pain starts without warning, it can be very alarming. The chart below identifies types of chest pain.

Chest pain

What to look for	Possible cause	Action
Severe central chest pain with shortness of breath and anxiety – relieved by rest	Angina	Help casualty to take any medicine, offer reassurance. If pain returns, treat as heart attack and call an ambulance.
Severe central chest pain not relieved by rest or angina medicines, possibly accompanied by sweating and nausea	Heart attack (see pages 126-127)	Give aspirin to chew and call an ambulance immediately.
Cold symptoms with cough and sharp one-sided chest pain on breathing in	Pleurisy (lung inflammation)	See a GP urgently.
Cold symptoms with cough and green sputum, fever	Chest infection	See GP as soon as possible.
Rash over one side of chest, stopping in midline	Shingles	Make appointment with GP.
Pain worse on bending, affected by food (made worse or better), possibly nausea.	Gastro-intestinal disorder	Make appointment with GP.

Childbirth

Sometimes babies arrive without much warning or too quickly to summon assistance. As long as there have been no problems in pregnancy, childbirth should occur naturally.

Stages of childbirth

Stage 1: Contractions of the uterus, increasing in frequency and intensity. This stage may last several hours.

Stage 2: The baby is born. This stage may last up to an hour.

Stage 3: The placenta (afterbirth) is expelled.

The first sign of labour is often a 'show' – the discharge of the mucus plug that has protected the cervix (entrance to the womb) throughout pregnancy. Another early sign can be the woman's waters breaking. This may cause merely a trickle or a fairly dramatic flood; what has happened is that the sac of amniotic fluid cushioning the baby has ruptured. Just before birth, the baby's head shows at the vaginal opening.

Action

1 Do nothing in stage 1 except to make the mother comfortable and offer any physical support, reassurance or other assistance she needs.
   At this stage there may be time to call for help.

2 Wash your hands thoroughly, including scrubbing under the nails. Wear disposable gloves if available

3 After the mother feels the urge to push, the baby's head should become visible at the vaginal opening.

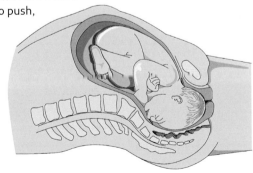

4 Allow the baby's head and shoulders to be pushed out, supporting the head gently with your hands. If the baby's face is covered by a thin skin or membrane, gently sweep this aside. If the umbilical cord is wrapped around the baby's neck, slip it carefully over the head.

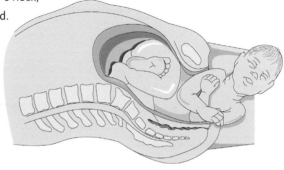

5 Gently lift the baby and lay him/her on the mother's abdomen with the head low to allow mucus to drain. Warning – newborn babies are slippery!

6 If the baby does not start breathing naturally, begin resuscitation (see pages 36–41).

7 Keep mother and baby warm until help arrives.

8 Up to half an hour after the birth, sometimes longer, the placenta will be expelled. Gentle massage of the lower part of the mother's tummy reduces bleeding. Collect the placenta in a clean container or plastic bag for examination later. The umbilical cord should be left uncut until help arrives.

9 Encourage the mother to put the baby to her breast.

10 Offer towels, a sanitary pad and warm water for washing.

When to call a doctor

▶ For a planned home birth, call the woman's midwife or doctor. If a hospital birth was planned, call an ambulance.

▶ If there is extensive bleeding or shock (see pages 149–150) call an ambulance at once.

▶ A woman having a miscarriage (see pages 142–143) needs urgent medical attention.

watch out!

▶ Do not urge the woman to push.
▶ Do not try to delay the birth.
▶ Do not tug or pull on the baby or the cord as they emerge.

Choking

Choking is very common, especially in babies and young children who tend to put things in their mouths and have a tiny airway, where small objects can easily get stuck.

Signs of choking

▶ victim may be unable to speak, may look panic-stricken
▶ signs of difficulty breathing
▶ clutching at throat, typically making a 'V' with hand on throat
▶ face and neck initially red, slowly turning blue

In a baby:

▶ strange noise, cannot cry properly
▶ face may turn blue

Action

1 If the person can understand, ask her to nod if she is choking.
2 Place yourself behind the victim with one arm around her middle and bend her forwards over your arm.
3 Give up to five vigorous slaps to the middle of her back with the flat of your other hand.

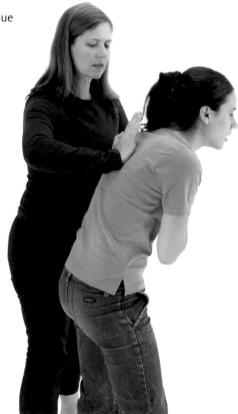

> **must know**
>
> Choking
> People are often embarrassed when they are choking - they may flee the room. If someone gets up from the dinner table in a hurry with possible choking symptoms, follow them to check.

4 If this does not work, make one hand into a fist and place it in the hollow underneath the rib cage above the naval.

5 Wrap your other hand over the first and grasp your wrist firmly.

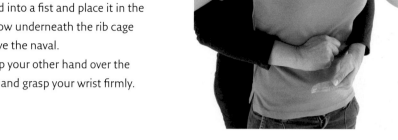

6 Give a short, sharp thrust upwards and inwards (towards yourself), then check whether this has dislodged the obstruction.

Repeat sequence up to three times if necessary. If you have no success in dislodging the obstruction, **call an ambulance**.

Keep repeating the sequence until the ambulance arrives or the airway is cleared.

Be prepared to perform resuscitation (see pages 38–41) if the victim becomes unconscious.

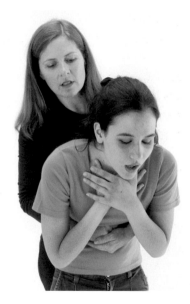

watch out!

Thrusts
▶ Never perform abdominal thrusts (into the tummy) unless someone is choking – you may cause serious injury.
▶ If the victim is **pregnant**, use chest thrusts (see page 92) not abdominal thrusts.

Choking in a child

The technique is very similar but uses chest thrusts first before abdominal thrusts.

1 Ask the child to cough.
2 If this fails to dislodge the obstruction, give up to five firm back slaps with the child bent forwards over one arm.

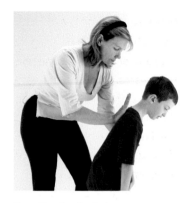

Up to five firm back slaps may dislodge the obstruction.

3 If this does not dislodge the obstruction, perform chest thrusts. Stand behind the child, place a clenched fist at the lower end of the child's breastbone, cover with your other hand and with both hands give a short, sharp pull upwards and inwards. Repeat up to five times.
4 If chest thrusts do not work, use abdominal thrusts as for an adult (see page 91). Place your fist between the lower end of the breast bone and the naval and pull sharply upwards and inwards, up to five times.
5 Repeat the sequence up to three times if necessary.
6 If you have no success, call an ambulance. Keep repeating the cycle until the ambulance arrives or the object is expelled. Be prepared to perform resuscitation (see pages 38–41) if the victim becomes unconscious.

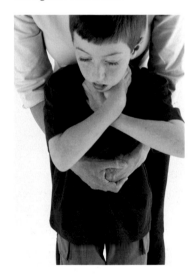

A short, sharp pull upwards with a clenched fist should be the next step.

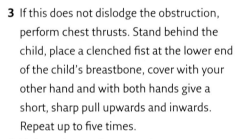

Choking in a baby

1 Lie the baby face-down along the length of your arm or across your knee with the head downwards.

2 Give up to five sharp slaps to the middle of the back, checking between each one to see if the obstruction has cleared.

3 If not, turn the baby face-up along your other arm or across your knee.

4 Use one finger to check for any obvious obstruction inside the mouth.

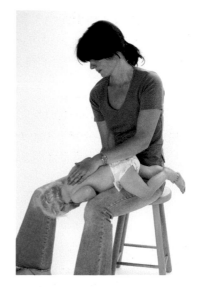

Make sure the baby is facing head downwards.

5 If nothing is found, place two fingertips on the lower end of the baby's breast bone and give up to five short, sharp chest thrusts, then check the mouth again.

6 Repeat the sequence up to three times. If the obstruction has not cleared, call an ambulance, taking the baby with you.

7 Keep repeating the cycle as necessary until the ambulance arrives. Be prepared to perform resuscitation (see page 41) if the baby becomes unconscious.

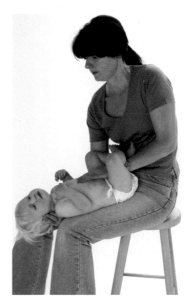

If the obstruction does not clear, call an ambulance immediately.

Collarbone, broken

A fractured collarbone is a common injury, usually resulting from a blow or fall on to the shoulder or a fall onto the outstretched hand.

The clavicles or collarbones join the shoulder blades to the breastbone, helping to support the arms. Most victims of a break are children and young people – fractured collarbone is often a sporting or riding injury.

Signs of a broken collarbone include:
▶ pain and swelling of the area
▶ pain increased by any movement of the arm on the affected side
▶ the casualty may support his arm at the elbow to relieve pain, or tilt his head towards that side
▶ the affected shoulder droops so it appears lower than the normal side
▶ reluctance to move affected limb
▶ obvious deformity if broken ends of bone are displaced
▶ nausea or vomiting

Action
1 Help the victim to sit down and ask him to support his elbow on the affected side with the other hand.
2 Loosen any items of clothing that may be adding to the discomfort, such as a tight collar or bra strap.

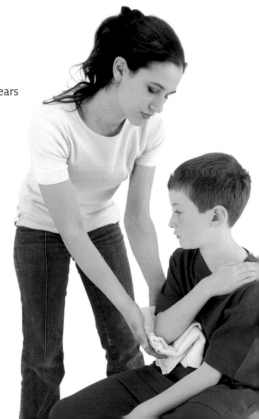

3 Gently place the affected arm diagonally across the chest, with the fingertips on the opposite shoulder.

4 Ask the casualty to move the elbow outwards slightly so that you can slip some soft padding – such as a folded towel or item of clothing – between his arm and chest wall. This should make him more comfortable.

5 Support the affected arm with an elevation sling (see page 71). If a sling is not available, improvise with a scarf or other piece of fabric.

6 Secure the sling in place with a broad bandage around the affected arm and the trunk – tie the knot over the arm on the uninjured side.

7 Arrange transport to hospital.

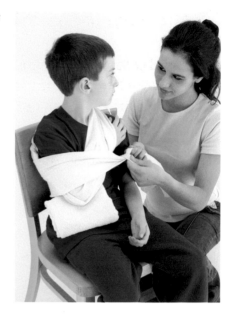

must know

It is important to seek urgent medical help for a broken bone. There is always a risk that a bone may move out of position and cause damage to blood vessels and organs.

Croup

Croup is an attack of breathing difficulty following respiratory infection in a baby or young child. It usually occurs at night and generally settles, but it can be frightening.

It is important to distinguish croup from an asthma attack (see page 74) or a very rare condition called epiglottitis – a potentially serious swelling of tissue at the back of the throat, which has similar symptoms.

Croup symptoms include a short, barking cough, in spasms, and a crowing or whistling noise on breathing in. In severe cases the child's lips and skin may appear bluish grey.

Action

1 Create a steamy atmosphere – run the hot tap or shower in the bathroom, or boil a kettle in the room (if you open the lid, the kettle will continue boiling and creating steam rather than cutting out – but make sure you don't let it boil dry).
2 Sit the child up on your knee and encourage steady breathing in the steam.
3 When the attack settles, put the child back to bed in a humid atmosphere – put a vaporiser near the bed – or place a wet towel on a radiator.
4 Call a doctor or ambulance if:
   ▸ breathing difficulty is severe or prolonged
   ▸ the child has a fever as well, especially if sitting bolt upright to breathe (these may indicate symptoms of epiglottitis)

Crush injury

A heavy object falling on top of someone may cause a variety of injuries including fractures and internal bleeding. Crush injuries often happen in building-site and road-traffic accidents.

If the person is pinned down under a heavy object, the crushing force may damage tissues and impair circulation to a limb. This causes tingling or numbness and probably pain, nausea and faintness.

In addition, toxins build up in the area. If the crushing force is suddenly removed, tissue fluid leaks into the area and shock (page 149) may develop. Even more dangerous, a sudden release of toxins into the circulation may cause kidney failure – so-called 'crush syndrome' – which can be fatal.

Action

1 Crush injuries are potentially very serious – always call an ambulance.

2 If the person has been crushed for less than 15 minutes, release them if possible. Treat associated injuries and call an ambulance.

3 If the person has been crushed for more than 15 minutes, do not attempt to move the object. Call an ambulance immediately, reassure and monitor the casualty, and be prepared to start resuscitation if necessary (see pages 36–41).

watch out!

Do not endanger yourself if there is a risk of other falling objects – call for help.

Do not attempt to remove a heavy object from a casualty. Releasing pressure from the damaged area may inflict further inury.

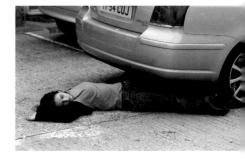

Diabetic incidents

Diabetes occurs because the body cannot produce sufficient insulin, the hormone that controls blood sugar levels. Some people with diabetes have to take insulin to regulate their blood sugar, and be very careful what and when they eat.

did you know?

At least a million people in the UK have diabetes and are not aware of it.

watch out!

If a person having a hypoglycaemic attack ('hypo') does not respond rapidly to sugar, or loses consciousness, call an ambulance.

must know

If someone with diabetes seems unwell and you are not sure whether his blood sugar is too high or too low, give sugar. This will rapidly correct dangerous hypoglycaemia and do little further harm in hyperglycaemia.

Too much insulin, or too little sugar, can cause blood sugar levels to drop dangerously low – a condition called hypoglycaemia. This is very serious and can rapidly cause unconsciousness and coma.

The opposite condition, too much blood sugar, is called hyperglycaemia. It also requires urgent treatment, but usually develops more slowly – over a period of hours or days rather than minutes – giving more time to get the person medical attention.

Some people with diabetes carry a card. However, a person may not be known to have diabetes.

Hypoglycaemia: signs and symptoms

Hypoglycaemia affects brain function; the symptoms occur rapidly and can be frightening. An attack is most likely to happen after a missed meal or too much insulin, but certain tablet treatments can also trigger a 'hypo'. Signs may include:

▶ faintness, giddiness, weakness or hunger
▶ shaking, trembling and palpitations
▶ pale, cold skin or sweating
▶ confusion or aggression – the person may appear drunk and even behave violently
▶ fits followed by the rapid onset of coma

Action

1 Help a conscious casualty to sit down. Give him some form of sugar – for instance, a sugary drink (try a carton of pure fruit juice), sugar lumps, sweets or chocolate. A person with diabetes may carry a sugar treatment, such as glucose gel.

2 If the person begins to recover, encourage him to eat a proper meal, drink and rest, and advise him to see his own doctor.

3 If the person is unconscious, call an ambulance. While waiting for help to arrive, check the victim's airway, breathing and circulation and start resuscitation if necessary (see pages 34–41). Put an unconscious but breathing casualty into the recovery position (see pages 42–43).

Hyperglycaemia: signs and symptoms

High blood sugar builds up over a long period of time, and can eventually lead to drowsiness and then coma. Before this, there may be a history of eating too much or taking too little insulin. The victim may have noticed some of the following symptoms: excessive urination; vomiting; warm, dry skin; an odour like pear drops or nail-varnish remover on his breath; and breathing problems or noisy breathing.

Action

1 Call an ambulance unless the person responds rapidly to sugar.

2 Monitor the casualty until help arrives, and be prepared to start resuscitation (see pages 36–41) if necessary.

want to know more?

For more information about living with diabetes, contact Diabetes UK. The organisation has an excellent website (www.diabetes.org.uk), or you can phone 020 7424 1000.

Diarrhoea and vomiting

Any type of irritation to the intestinal tract may cause diarrhoea or vomiting, or both. Causes include food poisoning, drugs or medicines, allergic reactions, poisoning and various medical conditions.

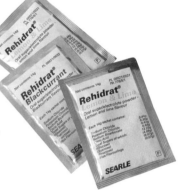

The most common danger is from dehydration – the person loses a lot of fluid, as well as vital salt and other minerals. This can have serious consequences, especially in babies and young children, the elderly, or people who are already ill.

Signs of illness may include diarrhoea or vomiting or both; abdominal pain; nausea and loss of appetite; and exhaustion after a prolonged episode. Sometimes, there is fever and sweating.

Treatment involves replacement of lost fluids and minerals – and attention to the cause of the problem.

Action

1 Make the casualty as comfortable as possible with access to a bathroom, a bucket if necessary and tissues, clean flannels and towels.

2 As soon as the casualty can tolerate fluids, encourage him or her to drink.

3 Give water, diluted fruit juice, weak slightly sweetened tea or, ideally, rehydration solutions – readily available over the counter or on prescription from chemists.

4 As soon as the person regains his or her appetite, offer bland, easily-digested snacks such as toast or soup – avoid spicy and acidic foods, fruit, high fibre foods such as beans and pulses, alcohol and tea or coffee for at least 24 hours.

watch out!

Never leave a casualty alone if her consciousness is fluctuating: an unconscious casualty may choke on inhaled vomit.

When to call a doctor

▶ Seek urgent medical advice if you suspect symptoms are due to an allergic reaction (see page 64), or poisoning (see page 146).

▶ Call a doctor if the condition does not ease within 48 hours, or if diarrhoea and/or vomiting are accompanied by severe pain, fever or other worrying symptoms.

▶ Call a doctor if the casualty is a baby or very young child who is not feeding.

▶ Elderly people, and those who are already ill or dehydrated are also at risk and need medical attention.

▶ Tell the casualty to talk to his or her own doctor if he or she suspects symptoms are related to any medication.

Women taking oral contraceptives

Any woman using oral contraceptives must not rely on her pill being absorbed and doing its job while she is unwell. It is important to use additional methods of contraception after a bout of severe diarrhoea both during recovery and for at least another week afterwards.

Rehydration solution

It is possible to make a rehydration solution using salt and sugar – one teaspoon salt and five teaspoons sugar dissolved in one litre of water. However, this is a last resort – if not made accurately, homemade solutions can be dangerous, especially for children.

watch out!

Dial 999 if you suspect symptoms are due to a severe reaction or poisoning.

did you know?

Cola is a good rehydration remedy for stomach upsets. Its acidity helps to kill *E. coli*, a bug that often causes food poisoning. Avoid excess wind by whisking out the bubbles before drinking.

Food poisoning

Diarrhoea and vomiting, often together, may occur after eating or drinking items contaminated with bacteria or viruses, or with the toxins produced by certain bacteria. Common sources include shellfish, processed meats, poultry that has been stored for too long or improperly thawed before cooking, and warm or cold cooked foods left out for any length of time. Produce from street vendors is particularly risky as hygiene precautions may not be adequate and equipment may not be properly cleaned.

► Symptoms can develop within hours of eating a contaminated food, or may be delayed – sometimes for several days.

► The general treatment is the same as for diarrhoea and vomiting (see above) – in other words fluid replacement and rest. If you are worried by the person's condition, or if the casualty is very young or very old, seek medical advice.

Avoiding 'traveller's diarrhoea'

► Wash your hands twice with soap before using them to put anything at all in your mouth, and dry your hands by air or a clean towel. If out and about, take antiseptic hand wipes with you.

► In high-risk areas avoid local drinking water or ice that has been made with it, dairy products and ice cream.

► Eat only fresh foods that have been properly heated through.

► Avoid salads washed in local drinking water.

► Avoid shellfish and fish that may have been on display unrefrigerated.

► Be aware that street food stalls may have doubtful hygiene standards.

► If possible, take a look in the restaurant kitchen: if it looks dirty or is swarming with flies, find somewhere else to eat.

Dizziness

Dizziness can make someone feel a sensation of movement, as if the ground is spinning, or as if he or she is swaying. It may also occur in susceptible people during car, ship or air journeys, and sometimes in acute anxiety or panic attacks.

Unpleasant symptoms may include a spinning or moving sensation, nausea or vomiting, possibly ringing in the ears or hearing loss, and sometimes pain or discharge from the ear.

did you know?

Dizziness is often part of an ear disorder, caused by disturbance to the tiny mechanisms in the inner ear that control balance.

Action

1 Help the casualty to sit or lie down.
2 A flow of fresh air or being fanned may help.
3 For travel sickness, encourage the casualty to gaze at the horizon.
4 Over-the-counter medications may help to prevent travel sickness, but they usually have to be taken in advance.
5 Travel sickness symptoms can persist for some time after the journey – stay with the casualty until he feels better.
6 Unless the cause is obvious – such as seasickness – advise the casualty to see her doctor.
7 Seek medical attention if there are any symptoms of an ear infection.

must know

If anyone in the household is affected by dizziness, and you have any gas appliances, there may be a fault and it could be emitting carbon monoxide. Switch the appliance off and get a professional to check.

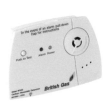

Drowning

Small children are the most likely victims of drowning, and they are at risk even in shallow water such as in a bath, paddling pool or pond.

Anyone falling into a lake, river or the sea around Britain is also at risk from hypothermia – even in summer. The shock of entering cold water may increase the danger and hamper efforts to swim to safety, even for experienced swimmers.

Danger signs of drowning
▶ someone struggling or in trouble in the water
▶ a body under the water or floating face-down on the surface
Once out of the water
▶ lack of breathing
▶ mottled, very pale or blue-tinged skin
▶ other signs of hypothermia – shivering, confusion, slow and shallow breathing, weak pulse

Action
1 If possible, reach out with your arms or throw something – such as a rope, pole or tree branch – for the victim to grasp. Then pull him out of the water.
2 Only enter the water if the person is out of reach or unconscious, and if you can do so without danger to yourself. Otherwise call for help.
3 If you must go into the water, stay on your feet and wade rather than swimming if at all possible.
4 Carry an unconscious person with his head down below chest level, so there is less risk of inhaling water.

5 Once out of the water, be prepared to
start resuscitation (see pages 36–41).
If the person is unconscious but breathing,
put him into the recovery position
(see pages 42–43).

6 Call an ambulance as soon as possible.

7 Shield the victim from the cold, remove
wet clothing and cover him with a blanket,
towels or clothing.

8 If necessary, treat for hypothermia
(page 133) while waiting for help to arrive.

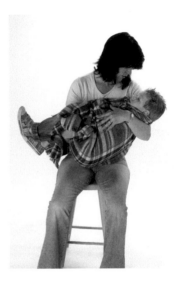

**Make sure you wrap up the victim well
so as to help to prevent or reverse the
effects of hypothermia.**

want to know more?

Keeping children safe around water
**Children love water and are irresistibly drawn to it. So it makes
sense to teach them how to behave near water. For more
information about teaching children to swim, contact the
Swimming Teachers' Association (STA). This UK-based charity has
an excellent website at www.sta.co.uk; telephone 01922 645097.
It aims 'to ensure that everyone gets the most out of swimming
safely, especially families with young children, the disabled and
keen kids'. It also provides comprehensive water-safety advice as
part of its Learn to Swim programme.**

Earache and ear problems

Earache is often due to an infection, either in the ear canal – common in swimmers – or in the middle ear. Children are most at risk of a middle ear infection, especially after a cold, and the pain may be severe.

did you know?

Dental problems such as tooth decay can cause earache. This is a type of 'referred pain'.

The most common ear problems tend to be due to an object getting stuck in the ear such as when small children accidentally insert a small button or a piece of food. It is also possible for an insect to get trapped inside the ear canal. Earwax may also be a problem when it becomes hard and encrusted. Whatever the cause, poking or proding in the ear is not advised as this can damage the skin lining the ear canal or the eardrum itself. Earache can also occur when flying, due to pressure changes in the middle ear.

Signs of ear problems may include:

▶ pain in the ear, or an unhappy infant holding or tugging ear on one side

▶ loss of hearing or ringing in the ear

▶ giddiness or dizziness

▶ a foreign body in the ear canal

▶ discharge from the ear

▶ sometimes, fever and being generally unwell – in infants, feeding or sleeping disturbances, irritability, vomiting or diarrhoea

must know

▶ Never plug a discharging ear – if necessary, cover the whole ear with a sterile pad until the victim reaches medical aid.

▶ Do not try to remove any foreign body from the ear – seek medical assistance.

Action

1 Give mild painkillers such as paracetamol or ibuprofen (do not give aspirin to children under 16).

2 A water bottle (warm not hot) wrapped in a towel and held over the ear may ease pain.

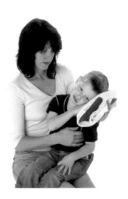

3 Pressure changes from flying may be relieved by making the ears 'pop' – close your mouth, hold your nose and 'blow' against the pressure.

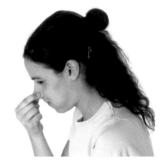

4 Trapped insects can often be cleared (or at least the alarming noise stopped) by flooding the ear canal with lukewarm water.

5 Call a doctor for:

▶ any severe earache in a child that persists for more than a few hours, or if earache is accompanied by fever, hearing loss or other symptom

▶ any ear problems in a baby under three months

watch out!

▶ Call a doctor urgently if a child with earache develops neck pain or stiffness or swelling.

▶ Seek urgent attention if there is blood or clear fluid draining from the ear, especially after any kind of head injury.

Electric shock

Accidents with domestic electricity are usually due to faulty wiring or appliances – such as a frayed flex or badly wired plug – or to unsafe handling, for example, changing a light bulb with wet hands.

Other common dangers are children attempting to poke objects into plug sockets, and adults mishandling power tools.

Signs of electric shock include unconsciousness, burns at the sites of entry and exit of the current, and difficulty breathing or no breathing. Call an ambulance at once.

Action

1 Do not touch a casualty who is still in contact with the current.

2 If possible, switch the electricity off at the mains and unplug the appliance.

3 If you cannot do this, you need to separate the casualty from the current without coming into contact with it yourself.

 ▸ Stand on some thick, insulating material, such as a block of wood or two telephone directories.

 ▸ Use a plastic or wood – not metal – pole, such as a broom handle to push the electrical equipment away from the casualty, or the casualty away from the power source.

 ▸ If you cannot do this, loop a length of rope around the casualty's arms or ankles and drag him clear that way, or as a last resort, tug on his clothing, being very careful not to touch his body – he may still be 'live'.

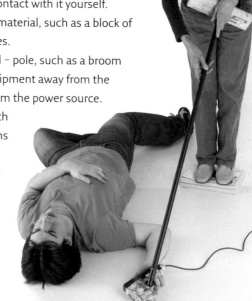

4 Check airway, breathing and circulation and be prepared to start resuscitation if necessary.

5 Place an unconscious but breathing casualty in the recovery position (see pages 42–43).

6 Treat any burns (see page 83–85) while awaiting the ambulance.

Eye injury

The eyes are vulnerable to injury through direct blows or scratches, foreign objects, chemical splashes and burns. Flying shards of metal or glass may penetrate the eye and leave little external sign.

Symptoms of an eye injury may include pain in the eye; blurred or lost vision; redness and watering; inability to open the eye; bruising around the eye (see black eye, page 77); a wound or bleeding near the eye; other signs of face injury (see page 112); or a foreign body visible in the eye. Any eye injury should be assessed by a doctor because of the potential for infection, scarring and loss of vision.

Action

For chemical splashes:

1 Ask the casualty to turn his head to one side and hold the eye open.
2 Flush with cold water, preferably under a tap, for 10 minutes. Ensure that the affected eye is lowermost, so that the other eye is not contaminated.
3 Hold or tape a sterile pad gently over the eye and seek urgent medical attention.

watch out!

Never touch anything sticking to the eye surface or embedded in the eyeball – take or send the victim to hospital.

For a small foreign body such as an eyelash or speck of dust:

1 Hold the eye open.

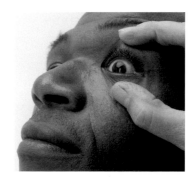

2 Flush it with water from a cup or tap, or with an eyewash solution. A towel over the casualty's shoulder will protect his clothes from water.

3 If this does not work, try to lift off the debris with the corner of a damp sterile swab or handkerchief.

4 If you do not succeed, or if pain persists – which may indicate scratching of the front of the eye – seek medical attention.

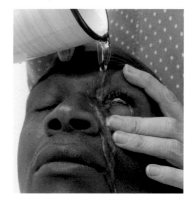

When to see a doctor

Any other eye injury requires immediate medical attention – do not attempt first aid. If possible, hold or tape a sterile pad across the eye. Ask the casualty to lie down on his back and to keep both eyes still: the eyes move together and any eye movement may cause pain and increase damage to the affected eye. In any penetrating eye injury, call an ambulance.

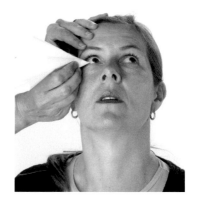

It may be possible to remove the debris with the corner of a damp, clean handkerchief.

Face injury

Facial injuries occur quite often. They may be as simple as a black eye (see page 77) or involve fractures, eye injuries or other serious damage. Facial injuries should always be looked at by a doctor, in case they are more serious than they appear.

Signs of facial injury may include pain, swelling, bruising or bleeding; difficulty speaking, swallowing or breathing; and visual disturbances. Look out for blood or fluid draining from the casualty's nose or ears – this may suggest a skull fracture.

Action

1 Check airway, breathing and circulation and be prepared to start resuscitation if necessary (see pages 34–41).

2 Call an ambulance for all but the most minor injury.

3 A cold compress (page 50) may help to reduce swelling.

4 Monitor and treat for shock (see pages 149-50) while awaiting medical help.

5 If the jaw is broken, support it with your hand, or ask the casualty to do so, on the way to hospital.

6 Call an ambulance immediately if the casualty has any difficulty breathing, fractures, an eye injury (see pages 110-111), or signs of head injury or concussion (see page 124).

watch out!

Never bandage the jaw or lower face – this can obstruct breathing or cause choking if the casualty vomits.

Fainting

Fainting occurs because of a temporary reduction of blood flow to the brain. The victim collapses, so boosting the flow, and the attack is self-limiting.

A person may faint after a prolonged period of standing, especially in a hot environment. Fainting can also be a reaction to pain, emotional trauma, exhaustion or hunger. Warning signs that someone might faint include giddiness, sweating and feeling light-headed; or a sense of nausea with sweating.

Action

1 If someone is about to faint, get him to sit or lie down - or at least cushion the fall if possible.
2 Raise the casualty's legs, to further improve blood flow to the brain.
3 Ensure a flow of fresh air.
4 Loosen tight clothing, especially around the neck and waist.
5 Offer reassurance and help the casualty to sit up slowly.

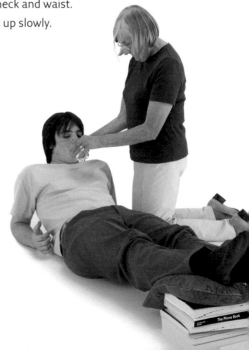

watch out!

If the casualty remains unconscious, or if recovery does not occur within a few minutes, call an ambulance.

Fever

A raised temperature – above the normal body temperature of about 37°C (98.6°F) – occurs in many infections, including common childhood illnesses.

must know

If a small child is very hot, use tepid (not cold) sponging to try to bring the temperature down.

Conditions such as colds, sore throat, earache or chickenpox, or local infections such as an abscess can all cause the temperature to go up. Signs of fever include:

▶ raised body temperature – if you don't have a thermometer, feel the forehead with your hand
▶ shivering and a 'chilled' feeling, with goosebumps or chattering teeth
▶ initially pale; later hot, with flushed cheeks and sweating
▶ sweating
▶ aches and pains
▶ headache

Fever is the body's normal response to infection and may help to fight invading germs. However, if the person is very uncomfortable, it is worth giving medicines to try to ease pain and inflammation and bring down the temperature.

Action

1 Put the person to bed with a light covering, or let him rest in a well-ventilated room.

watch out!

Never give painkillers containing aspirin to a child under 16.

2 Give plenty of cool fluids to drink.
3 Give mild painkillers such as paracetamol or ibuprofen (not aspirin for children under 16) if the casualty is very uncomfortable.
4 Treat any obvious associated conditions, such as earache (see pages 106–107).

5 If a small child is very hot, use tepid (not cold) sponging to try to bring the temperature down, as long as this does not make the child more uncomfortable.

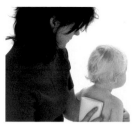

6 Watch for the danger signs of heat stroke (see pages 128–129), meningitis (see pages 140–141) or febrile convulsions (see page 117).

7 Monitor the casualty's temperature and general condition every ten minutes.

Should you call a doctor?

▶ If you suspect meningitis, heat stroke or febrile convulsions, call an ambulance.

▶ Call your doctor if a child's temperature rises above 40°C (104°F).

▶ Seek medical advice if you are at all concerned about the casualty's condition – phone NHS Direct on 0845 46 47.

▶ Always inform a doctor if fever follows a recent trip abroad.

Taking a child's temperature

There are several different ways of taking a child's temperature. Using a thermometer strip that you put on the child's forehead is the easiest way – but it isn't very accurate. A digital or mercury thermometer placed under the arm gives a better reading, but this will be 0.6°C (0.9F) lower than the true temperature.

If you are worried about your baby or child's temperature, call NHS Direct on 0845 46 47 for advice. You will usually be able to tell whether your child has a temperature simply by touching his or her forehead.

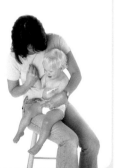

Fits

A fit, also called a seizure or convulsion, can be very alarming to witness, especially if it occurs unexpectedly. Try to remain calm and keep any hazardous items away from the casualty.

did you know?

A fit is caused by a disturbance of electrical activity in the brain.
It usually results in uncontrolled movements and impaired consciousness.

Fits may be the result of disease, injury or epilepsy. Most victims make a full recovery. The important action for any bystander is to protect the person from injury during the fit.

Signs of a fit include sudden unconsciousness – the person often utters a cry or roar and falls to the floor. There may also be arching of the back; convulsive twitching and jerking of the limbs; clenched jaw, sometimes foaming at the mouth; and noisy or absent breathing with blue lips. Sometimes, there is a loss of bladder or bowel control. After a few minutes, the muscles relax and the casualty comes round, but is usually dazed for a while and may wish to sleep.

Action

1 If someone is about to collapse, try to cushion the fall.

2 Take away any hazardous items such as glasses or knives.

3 Move dangerous objects out of the person's path so he cannot hurt himself while fitting.

4 If he has fallen near heavy furniture or other objects that cannot be moved, place cushions or other padding around the objects to prevent further injury.

5 Once the fit has stopped place a pad under his head and loosen any tight clothing around his neck.

watch out!

▶ Never try to restrain the person's movements or insert anything between his teeth.

▶ Do not move the person unless to prevent danger (such as falling into water).

6 Call an ambulance if the casualty:
- ▶ fits for more than five minutes
- ▶ is injured
- ▶does not regain consciousness within 10 minutes

7 When fitting stops, check the airway and breathing and be prepared to start resuscitation if necessary (see pages 34–41).

8 Call a doctor if this is the person's first fit.

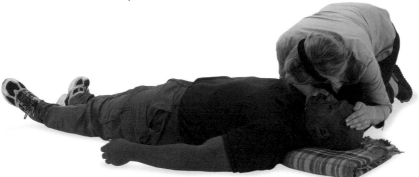

Febrile convulsions in children

Children under the age of four are at risk of fits developing when they have a raised temperature. Febrile convulsions are very alarming, but rarely dangerous.

Symptoms include:
- ▶ feverish, flushed, hot child
- ▶ eyes rolled upwards, fixed or crossed
- ▶ jerking limbs, arched back, stiffness, clenched fists

Action

1 Position soft padding around the child to avoid injury.

2 Remove clothing and cool the child (see pages 114-115).

3 Call an ambulance if this is the child's first fit.

Frostbite

Frostbite occurs when an extremity gets so cold that the tissues actually freeze. It most often occurs in the hands or feet, but the tip of the nose and earlobes can also be affected.

watch out!

Do not rub the affected part – you may damage the tissue more.

Signs of frostbite include, to begin with, pale skin on the fingers, toes or other extremity; pins and needles, progressing to numbness; and hard, stiff skin. Later, the skin colour changes from white to mottled blue. In severe cases, frostbite can cause permanent damage and gangrene: if gangrene develops, the skin turns black. On rewarming, the skin often becomes red, hot and painful and may blister.

Action

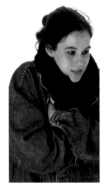

1 If possible, get the casualty into the warm.

2 Handle the affected part very gently.

3 Remove any constrictions such as gloves, boots and rings.

4 Gently warm the affected area with warm (not hot) water – about 40°C (104°F). If there is no water, use your hands. If a person's hands are affected, ask her to tuck her hands into her armpits.

5 Ensure the affected area is dry and apply a bandage dressing.

6 Check for associated hypothermia and treat accordingly (see page 122)

7 Seek medical attention as soon as possible.

did you know?

Tissue damage from frostbite is due to ice crystals forming in the cells, then expanding, and rupturing them.

want to know more?

Who is most vulnerable to frostbite?
People with circulation problems, those who have been drinking alcohol, and anyone taking certain medications – such as beta-blockers for heart disease – should be careful in the cold. Wear several layers of clothes, and a warm hat, gloves, socks and boots.

Gas or smoke inhalation

Inhaling gases or smoke can be fatal. Apart from the direct toxic effects of poisonous fumes, victims may suffocate (page 161) because insufficient oxygen reaches their lungs.

The most likely form of poisonous gas inhalation is carbon monoxide. This is usually due to faulty maintenance of heaters and flues, or to car exhaust fumes building up in the confined space of a garage. Most people killed in house fires die from smoke inhalation. Smoke may also contain poisonous fumes from burning synthetic materials.

Signs of poison inhalation include:
▶ grey-blue skin, possibly red-tinged in carbon monoxide poisoning
▶ difficult or noisy breathing
▶ coughing or wheezing
▶ headache
▶ confusion
▶ impaired consciousness

Action
1 Call an ambulance immediately, and the fire brigade if appropriate.
2 If it is possible to do so safely, get the victim into fresh air. If entering a room or garage filled with fumes, open doors and windows wide first.
3 Check breathing and circulation and start resuscitation if necessary (see pages 34-41).
4 Place an unconscious but breathing casualty into the recovery position (see pages 42-43) while awaiting help.
5 Treat any burns or other injuries.

must know

Do not try to rescue casualties if this means endangering yourself – call for help instead.

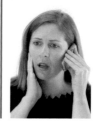

Hand injury

The hand may be injured by punching, crushing, falls or wounding. Broken bones, dislocations and sprains of the fingers, and tendon or nerve injuries are possible.

Signs of hand injury include pain; restricted movements at knuckles and finger joints; swelling and bruising; a bleeding wound; and deformity if there is a fracture or dislocation – compare the injured hand with the other one.

All hand injuries should be regarded as potentially serious because of the risk of long-term complications.

did you know?

Dislocated finger If a finger is dislocated, bandage as shown in the illustrations, taking care not to apply any pressure – you could damage nerves or blood vessels. Loosen the bandage if the casualty complains of pins and needles or numbness in the fingertips.

Action

1 Remove any bracelets or rings, in case the hand or fingers swell.

2 Place a sterile dressing or clean pad over any wound.

3 Put padding around the hand – cotton wool or any soft material – and secure it in place.

4 Bandage around the hand. Start by laying the hand on the base of a triangular bandage and fold the point of the bandage down over the fingers, covering the injured area.

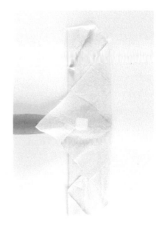

5 Cross the ends of the bandage around the wrist.

6 Tie ends together with a secure knot. Then pull the point of the bandage up over the knot and tuck it in to hold the bandage in place. Add tape or a safety pin to secure in place if necessary.

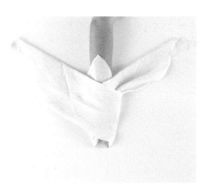

7 Raise the hand above the level of the heart.

8 Gently place the affected arm across the casualty's chest with the fingertips to the opposite shoulder – ask the casualty to support the elbow of the affected arm, if possible.

9 Support the arm in an elevation sling (see pages 56–57), and strap to the chest with a broad bandage if necessary.

10 Seek medical advice for all but the most trivial hand injury, as any damage to the nerves, tendons or blood vessels could impair hand movement and cause long-term disability. Take or send the casualty to hospital.

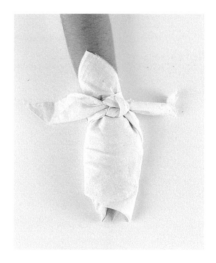

Wounds to the palm

Wounds to the palm may bleed profusely. There is particular risk of injury to the tendons or nerves controlling finger movement, or to the nerves that supply the crucial sensations of the fingertips.

Action

1 If there is profuse bleeding, watch for signs of shock (see pages 149-150) and treat accordingly.
2 Place a sterile dressing or clean pad against the wound.
3 Ask the casualty to make a fist to press against the pad. If he finds it difficult to exert pressure, ask him to press with the uninjured hand.
4 Bandage the fist in this position.
5 Place the affected arm across the casualty's chest and support the arm in an elevation sling (see pages 56-57).
6 Take or send the casualty to hospital.

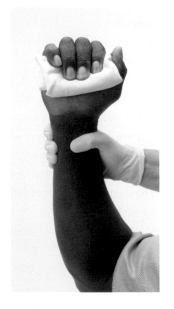

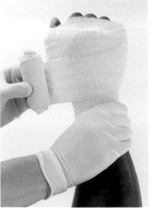

watch out!

If there is a foreign object embedded in a palm wound, do not attempt to remove it – pad around it until you can bandage on top.

Headache and migraine

Headaches are extremely common, and usually get better on their own or with rest and supportive treatment. An excruciating headache along with other symptoms occurs in migraine.

Headaches may result from stress and tension, an infection – especially if there is a raised temperature, drinking excess alcohol, certain drugs or medicines, or poisoning. Some people suffer from migraine attacks, which can cause very specific symptoms along with an agonising headache.

Rarely, headache is associated with serious conditions such as stroke (see page 160) or meningitis (see pages 140-141).

Headache and migraine symptoms include feeling miserable with pain in the head; nausea or vomiting – especially in migraine; and associated visual disturbances in migraine.

watch out!

Never give aspirin-containing painkillers to a child under 16.

Action

1 Seek urgent medical attention if there has been a head injury (see page 124) or if you suspect meningitis (page 140).
2 Otherwise, help the casualty to lie down in a quiet room.
3 Offer a cold compress for the forehead.
4 Give mild painkillers if the casualty wants them.
5 Advise the casualty to seek medical advice if symptoms are severe, persistent or unusual.

want to know more?

The Migraine Action Association (www.migraine.org.uk) can help migraine sufferers to identify their trigger factors and recognise early warning signs. It provides information on long established treatments as well as the latest developments in both conventional and complementary medicine.

Head injury

Any head injury is potentially serious because of the risk of skull fracture or damage to the brain. There is also a risk of associated neck and spinal injury.

A head injury can trigger bleeding or swelling inside the skull, which may cause compression of the brain and possibly life-threatening complications. There may be spinal injury as well.

Concussion can follow a fall or blow to the head, or a fall onto the buttocks, transmitting forces up the spine. The brain is shaken inside the skull, causing brief loss of consciousness. On recovery there may be a temporary mild headache, dizziness and loss of short-term memory – especially for events leading up to the accident. If someone who has been concussed develops new symptoms, there may be a more serious injury.

The scalp is richly supplied with blood vessels, so minor knocks often cause dramatic bumps (see page 82), and head wounds may bleed profusely. Indeed, bleeding often looks more alarming than it really is. However, care must always be taken not to miss a serious underlying injury.

Signs of severe head injury

Symptoms may include severe headache, nausea or vomiting and the person could appear confused, disorientated or not quite 'with it'. There may be irritability and loss of coordination. Other danger signs are:

▶ blood or fluid draining from the ears

▶ blurred or double vision

▶ unequal pupil size

▶ weakness or paralysis of one side of the body

▶ difficult, slow or noisy breathing

▶ unconsciousness or coma

watch out!

Do not move an unconscious casualty unless absolutely necessary.

Action

Call an ambulance at once if the victim does not respond
to simple commands or has any of the signs of severe head
injury described above.

If the casualty is unconscious, handle the head very
carefully, as for spinal injury (see pages 152–154).

1 Use the jaw-thrust method (see page 154) to open the airway.
2 Treat any scalp wounds:
   ▶ replace any flaps of skin
   ▶ apply a sterile dressing
   ▶ if bleeding continues, apply firm pressure
     with a pad on top of the dressing
   ▶ secure the dressing with a roller or triangular bandage
3 Apply an ice pack (see page 50) to any bumps or bruises on the scalp.
4 Monitor the casualty extremely carefully, watching
   especially for deterioration of consciousness.
5 Watch for and treat signs of shock (page 149–150).
6 Monitor breathing and circulation and be prepared to start
   resuscitation if necessary (pages 34–41).
7 If there is an open wound, take or send
   the casualty to hospital.
8 Advise any casualty who has been concussed to seek hospital
   attention at once if further symptoms develop.

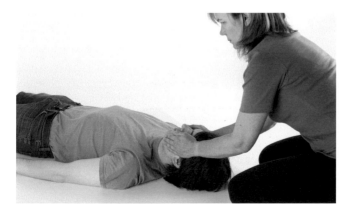

must know

**Suspected neck
injury**
If there is a head
injury, you should
always suspect the
possibility of a
neck or spinal
injury, too. Tell the
casualty not to
move. Place your
hands on either
side of his head to
keep the head,
neck and spine
stable and aligned.

Heart attack

A heart attack occurs when one of the arteries supplying the heart with blood becomes blocked, usually due to a blood clot. The heart cannot pump properly due to the loss of oxygen supply and the part of the heart muscle supplied by that artery may be damaged.

watch out!

Dial 999 at once. Do not delay seeking help – the earlier treatment is given, the better the victim's chance of survival.

When someone is having a heart attack the priority is to get him or her to a hospital. Early treatment in hospital with clot-dissolving drugs can be life-saving and prevent long-term complications.

Signs of a heart attack

▶ severe pain in centre of chest that may spread to jaw or arms, especially the left arm

▶ pain may be described as crushing or vice-like

▶ unlike angina pain, it does not ease with rest

▶ pain or discomfort in upper abdomen

▶ breathlessness, dizziness or faintness

Look after your heart

According to the British Heart Foundation (visit www.bhf.org.uk) there are five steps that everyone could take to benefit their heart.

1 Healthy eating: cut down on saturated fats in red meat, cakes, chips and dairy products and eat more fish, poultry and vegetables.

2 Be more active: half an hour a day – even simply walking – makes all the difference and this can be included in your daily routine.

3 Be smoke free: when you quit smoking, the risk of heart attack starts to reduce and it is halved after just a year of stopping.

4 Reduce alcohol: binge drinking increases your risk of having another heart attack. Drink in moderation.

5 Trim excess weight: eating a balanced diet, drinking alcohol in moderation and becoming more physically active will help you to lose weight and maintain a healthy body and heart.

- pale skin; profuse sweating
- grey, clammy appearance, with blue-tinged lips
- nausea or vomiting
- anxiety, sense of impending doom
- collapse, unconsciousness.

Action

1 Call an ambulance at once – tell the operator that you suspect a heart attack.
2 Sit the person down in a position they find comfortable – often with the head, shoulders and knees supported.
3 Be calm and reassuring – anxiety and panic increase stress on the heart.
4 Give a conscious casualty a standard aspirin tablet to chew and then swallow (not swallow whole) and ask him to do so slowly.
5 If the person usually takes medication for angina, help him to take that as well.
6 Monitor breathing and circulation while awaiting help. Be prepared to start resuscitation if necessary (pages 36–41). Place an unconscious casualty who is breathing in the recovery position (see pages 42–43).

must know

Give aspirin
- Straightaway give a standard 300mg aspirin tablet (or four of the low-dose tablets that many people take daily to prevent heart disease).
- Do not give any food or drink.

Call an ambulance immediately and make it clear that you suspect a heart attack.

Heat exhaustion and heat stroke

Heat exhaustion occurs when an excessive loss of salt and water through perspiration leads to dehydration. Heat stroke is a failure of the body's 'thermostat' resulting in dangerous overheating.

Heat exhaustion is due to a gradual overload of the body's mechanisms for heat regulation, which can happen when people are suddenly exposed to a much hotter climate than they are used to. Those who are already dehydrated due to diarrhoea or vomiting are especially at risk.

Heat stroke may follow heat exhaustion, or it may occur during over-exertion in hot conditions, or it may be the result of an illness causing fever. In heat stroke, sweating stops – so the body can no longer be cooled by sweat evaporation – while the 'thermostat' in the brain fails, causing body temperature to rise to life-threatening levels. It requires urgent treatment to stop damage to vital organs and even death.

must know

Drug danger
It is important to realise that both heat exhaustion and heat stroke can occur with use of drugs, such as Ecstasy, when combined with over-exertion in hot conditions.

Spot the difference

Early signs of both heat exhaustion and heat stroke are similar: the victim may seem restless, dizzy or confused and develop a sudden headache.

▶ If the person is sweating, looks pale and clammy, and feels nauseous or is experiencing cramps, suspect heat exhaustion.

▶ In heat stroke there is no sweat – instead the skin is hot, flushed and dry. The person has a fever and may collapse.

Action for heat exhaustion

1 Lie the casualty down somewhere cool, preferably with a breeze or fan.
2 Raise the legs.
3 Encourage the casualty to take frequent sips of cool water.
4 Then offer a rehydrating solution (available from pharmacies) if possible, or, as a last resort, a very weak salt solution (one level teaspoon of salt in one litre of water).
5 Anyone who has had heat exhaustion should be checked by a doctor even after apparent recovery. An affected child should be seen urgently.

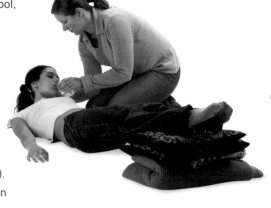

Action for heat stroke

1 Call an ambulance.
2 Remove clothing and wrap the casualty in a wet sheet.
3 Keep the sheet cool and wet and fan the casualty until his temperature falls.
4 Once the temperature has returned to normal, replace the wet sheet with a dry one – but be prepared to start cooling again if the temperature rises again.
5 Be prepared to start resuscitation if necessary (pages 36–41). Place an unconscious casualty in the recovery position (see pages 42–43).

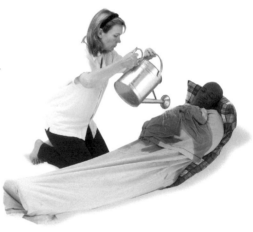

watch out!

Dial 999 at once if you suspect heat stroke. It can develop very quickly and without warning. There may be rapid deterioration and cooling is urgent – do not delay treatment.

Hip and pelvic injury

The most common form of hip injury is a fracture of the neck of the femur (thigh bone) within the hip joint. The pelvis itself is usually injured by an indirect force such as a crushing injury.

Hip fractures tend to occur after a fall, particularly in elderly women with osteoporosis (bone thinning), for whom this injury is a major cause of disability.

The pelvis may be damaged by crushing or an impact on the knee that forces the head of the femur back through the hip joint, as may occur in a car crash. Pelvic injuries are often very serious due to associated damage to blood vessels, nerves and nearby organs.

What to look for
Hip and pelvic injuries share several symptoms. These may include:
▶ severe pain, which increases with movement
▶ inability to stand or walk
▶ nausea, faintness or giddiness
▶ pale, clammy skin
▶ signs of shock (see page 149) from internal bleeding
▶ swelling and bruising

In a hip fracture:
▶ knee and foot on the affected side may be turned outwards
▶ the affected leg may appear shorter than the other side

In a fractured pelvis:
▶ there may be bleeding from the urethra (urine outlet)

Action: hip fracture

1 Help the casualty to lie down and place some support alongside the leg, such as a folded blanket.
2 Gently try to straighten the affected leg by pulling steadily in the line of the bone, but stop if this causes severe pain.
3 Call an ambulance.
4 While awaiting the ambulance, immobilise the leg by splinting it to the other leg as shown, right.
5 Treat shock if it develops (see pages 149–150) but do not raise the legs.

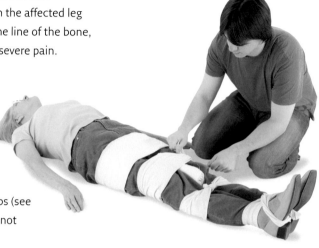

Action: pelvic injury

1 Help the casualty to lie down.
2 Support the legs with padding in a position that the casualty finds comfortable – straight and flat or with the knees slightly bent upwards.
3 Bandage the legs together to stop them from moving, starting with the ankles and then doing the knees (right). Stop if this causes pain.
4 Call an ambulance.
5 Treat shock if it develops (see pages 149–150) but do not raise the legs.

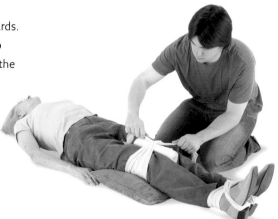

Hyperventilation

Hyperventilation means overbreathing. It may occur as an overreaction to any physical or emotional shock or stress in a susceptible individual.

Hyperventilation is also a feature of panic attacks – sudden intense fear provoked by a particular object or situation.

Affected people show extreme anxiety or fear, with loss of control. Overbreathing causes too much carbon dioxide to be blown out, which triggers further symptoms.

Signs of hyperventilation may include rapid breathing, dizziness or faintness, trembling or tingling in the fingers, and crying, screaming or dramatic language and gestures.

Action

1 Speak kindly but firmly, and offer reassurance.
2 If possible, take the person to a quiet place away from any audience. If not, ask onlookers to leave.
3 Ask the person to hold a paper bag over the mouth and nose and breathe in and out of it.
4 Do this in cycles of 10 breaths into the bag followed by a 15-second break, for as long as necessary.
5 Suggest the person talks to his or her doctor about controlling future hyperventilation or panic attacks.

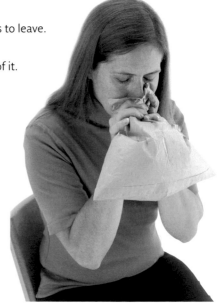

watch out!

Do not slap the person's face.

Hypothermia

Hypothermia occurs when the core body temperature falls below 35°C (95°F). If the temperature continues to fall, organs may stop working and the condition becomes life-threatening.

Hypothermia may occur in drowning victims (see pages 104–105) or in people trapped outside in cold conditions. Children lose body heat more easily than adults so are at higher risk from exposure. Older people in poorly heated homes are especially vulnerable as their bodies adapt less well to cold conditions and they may develop hypothermia slowly over several days.

Exposure to cold is estimated to cause 30,000 deaths a year in the UK. The charity Age Concern estimates that every time the temperature drops one degree Celsius below average, about 8,000 more elderly people will die.

Signs of hypothermia include:

▶ shivering
▶ cold, pale, dry skin
▶ confusion, lethargy or slurred speech
▶ slow, shallow breathing
▶ slow, weak pulse
▶ unconsciousness

Action: if outside

1 Protect the victim from further cold – find or improvise shelter.
2 Remove wet clothing from the victim and cover with dry blankets or clothes.
3 Insulate the victim from cold ground by placing material padding underneath.

must know

Keep children warm
Children are at risk of hypothermia, especially when waiting for school trains or buses in cold, wet weather. If it's windy too, be aware that wind makes cold more chilling. Children will stay warmer if they wear several layers along with hats, mittens, coats and waterproof boots. Make sure they eat properly.

4 Shout for help and dial 999 for an ambulance.
5 While awaiting help, lie next to the victim and use your body heat to help keep him or her warm.
6 Do not give the person any alcohol or cigarettes.
7 Be prepared to start resuscitation if necessary (see pages 36–41).

Action: if inside
1 Gradually warm the victim with layers of blankets and sips of warm liquids while awaiting medical help. **Do not** use a hot bath, fire or heater or hot-water bottle.
2 Do not give the person any alcohol or cigarettes.
3 Be prepared to start resuscitation if necessary (see pages 36–41).
4 Call a doctor: the person may have other medical problems that made him or her vulnerable to hypothermia.

watch out!

Slowly does it
Never warm someone with hypothermia too quickly. Avoid hot baths, fires and other heaters.

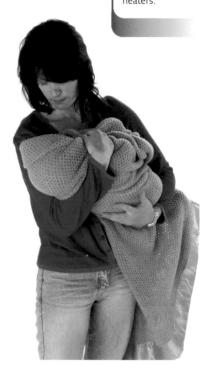

want to know more?

Age Concern runs a 'Be a Good Neighbour' scheme in winter, which asks people to be aware of elderly people living nearby. This can be as simple as popping in for a chat, or assisting with small jobs – from picking up a prescription to clearing a snowy path. For details, call Age Concern's freefone line on 0800 00 99 66.

Indigestion

Indigestion is very common and usually not serious. Simple measures, such as avoiding large meals, spicy foods and alcohol, especially before bedtime, can help to prevent indigestion.

Signs of indigestion include stomach ache, a sense of fullness or bloating, belching or nausea, and symptoms that come and go.

Action

1 Over-the-counter antacids may help to relieve symptoms.

2 Offer a hot-water bottle wrapped in a towel to place on the stomach.

3 Dial 999 if the pain is very severe, moves to the chest, jaw or arms, or is accompanied by vomiting, sweating, passing blood or black stools, or feeling very unwell.

4 Seek advice if an attack lasts for more than three hours, or interferes with eating or sleeping.

Hiccups

Hiccups are due to spasm of the diaphragm, sometimes caused by swallowing air, or by too much alcohol. Any of these tricks may stop an attack – though they are not all scientifically proven:

▶ hold your breath

▶ breathe in and out of a paper bag for 60 seconds (never put a plastic bag over the face)

▶ sip water from the 'wrong' side of a glass

▶ place a teaspoon of sugar towards the back of the tongue

must know

If an indigestion problem is getting worse or more frequent, or is accompanied by weight loss, difficulty in swallowing or other symptoms, talk to a doctor.

watch out!

Do not ignore persistent or severe pain or other symptoms: sometimes indigestion indicates an underlying disease.

Intoxication

Drug and alcohol intoxication can be dangerous not only in terms of the physical and psychological effects but also because of the increased risk of accidents.

People under the influence of drugs or alcohol may be clumsy and uncoordinated, and their judgment may be impaired: they often do things that they later regret, including engaging in unwise sexual liaisons.

Types of drugs include:

▶ narcotics – sedative properties
▶ stimulants – produce excitement, increase heart and breathing rate
▶ hallucinogens (including Ecstasy) – mind-altering
▶ cannabis – produces euphoria plus a sense of relaxation

What to look for

Symptoms vary with the type of drug and stage of intoxication. Any drug, including alcohol, is potentially fatal in overdose (see page 145). Signs of intoxication include:

▶ altered mood – excited, tearful, paranoid or aggressive
▶ loss of inhibitions – grandiose behaviour and gestures, inappropriate sexual behaviour, violent or criminal acts
▶ staggering, slurred speech, incoherence
▶ nausea, vomiting
▶ dizziness, faintness
▶ altered pupils – pinpoint, dilated or unreactive (not contracting to light)
▶ drowsiness and confusion, or alertness and agitation
▶ delusions, hallucinations
▶ rapid breathing or slow, shallow breathing
▶ tremors or convulsions

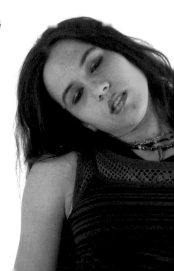

Dehydration can also occur with intoxication, especially when Ecstasy is combined with energetic dancing in a hot club atmosphere. Dehydration has its own danger signs, including headache, dizziness, sudden tiredness, muscle cramps and vomiting. There will probably be an inability to sweat and poor or absent urine output. Eventually, consciousness is impaired and the person may collapse and fall into a coma.

Action

1 Help a conscious person to a safe, comfortable place.
2 Lie a conscious casualty on his or her side – this will help to prevent choking if the casualty vomits.
3 Call a doctor if you are worried about the person's condition.
4 Get help if the person is aggressive or violent, or if he or she needs medical assistance.
5 Call an ambulance if the person collapses, becomes unconscious, is unrousable, has difficulty breathing or starts to fit.
6 Put an unconscious but breathing casualty into the recovery position (see pages 42–43).
7 Stay with the person and monitor his or her breathing. Be prepared to start resuscitation if necessary (pages 34–41).
8 If intoxication is part of a long-term drug or alcohol problem, encourage the person to seek help.

(see pages 42–43).

must know

What not to do
▶ Don't allow the person to drive.
▶ Don't give food or drink – you may encourage vomiting and choking. The **exception** is – Ecstasy: take the person somewhere cool and give non-alcoholic fluids.
▶ Don't give any medicines – there could be harmful drug interactions.
▶ Don't argue with or question an intoxicated person.
▶ Don't confront the person until he or she has sobered up.

Spotting drug use in teenagers – and getting help

▶ Parents should be on the lookout for altered behaviour – such as withdrawal or aggression; lying or stealing; impaired family relationships; decreased school performance; new friends or friends who use drugs; staying out late or running away; and getting into trouble with the law.
▶ Anyone worried about their own or someone else's drug use can 'talk to Frank', a free, confidential drugs helpline which provides advice, information and support to anyone concerned about drug and solvent misuse.
▶ Helpline: 0800 77 66 00 (manned seven days a week, 24 hours)
Website: www.talktofrank.com

Leg and knee injury

The bones of the leg can be broken by impact, twisting or direct blows. Knees are commonly injured in sporting accidents and falls.

must know

Get it looked at
Always seek medical help, as without prompt treatment there is a risk of impaired mobility.

The femur or thighbone is the strongest bone in the body and it takes considerable force to fracture it along its length (although a fracture of the neck of the femur within the hip joint is quite common, see page 130). This most often occurs after a fall from a great height, or a severe impact such as a car accident.

There are two bones in the lower leg, the tibia and the fibula. The tibia is most often broken by a heavy blow, sometimes producing an open wound. The fibula is thinner and can be broken by the kind of twisting that may cause a sprained ankle (see page 156).

Symptoms of serious leg injury include pain, bruising, deformity, difficulty walking or inability to walk, and swelling, especially at the knee.

The knee joint is quite complicated and may be damaged by direct force or violent twisting movements. Injuries from sporting incidents, falls and other accidents are common. There may be a sprain, damage to the knee cartilage or a fracture of the kneecap (patella). A serious knee injury will cause locking of joint, extreme pain on attempting to straighten it, and difficulty in bending the joint.

watch out!

▶ never attempt to straighten a knee joint by force
▶ do not give the casualty any food or drink, as an anaesthetic may be needed

Action

1 Help the casualty to lie down.
2 Treat any open wounds (see pages 164–167).
3 Support the legs with padding in a position that the casualty finds comfortable.
4 Call an ambulance.

Suspected fractures

1 Immobilise the legs, using the uninjured leg to splint the broken one.
2 Bring the uninjured leg to the side of the injured one.
3 Slide bandages under both legs at the ankles and knees, and above and below the suspected fracture site.

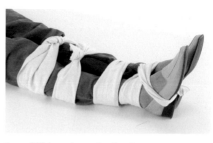

Immobilising a lower leg fracture

4 Place padding between the lower legs for comfort.
5 Roll bandage in a figure of eight around the feet and ankles.
6 Tie the bandages with the knots on the uninjured side, but stop if this causes pain.

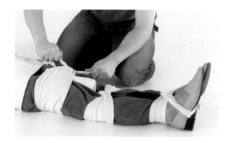

Immobilising a thigh fracture

Possible fracture near ankle

Wrap one bandage around the feet and a separate one around the legs just above the ankle instead of using a figure of eight.

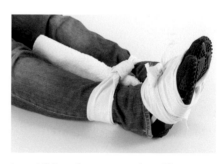

Immobilising a fracture near the ankle

Knee injuries

1 Wrap soft padding around the knee joint.
2 Bandage the legs together from mid-thigh to mid-calf, to stop the knee from moving.

Meningitis

Meningitis is a potentially serious condition in which the membranes surrounding the brain and spinal cord become inflamed, due to infection with one of a number of bacteria or viruses. Always call a doctor if you suspect meningitis.

Meningitis can occur at any age but children and young people are especially vulnerable. Unfortunately, the symptoms often mimic those of other common childhood illnesses.

With prompt treatment most people make a full recovery, but delayed recognition is common and without treatment there may be complications. These can include deafness and brain damage. Meningitis can even be fatal – so seek medical attention urgently if you suspect it.

When to suspect meningitis
Symptoms vary but may include:
▶ high temperature
▶ vomiting
▶ severe headache
▶ neck pain or stiffness (cannot touch chin to chest)

must know

The rash of meningitis
The rash that often accompanies meningitis typically occurs as clusters of small red or purple spots that look a bit like bruising. Unlike the spots of most rashes, these do not fade under pressure – so the classic test is to press the skin with the side of a glass. If the spots do not fade but are still clearly visible through the glass, the person may have meningitis and needs urgent medical attention.

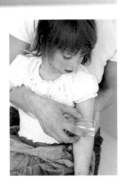

- dislike of the light – may say that light hurts the eyes
- confusion
- seizures
- skin rash

In babies and young children:
- high-pitched cry
- drowsiness or restlessness
- loss of interest in feeding

    Do not expect all these signs: people with the disease may not display all the symptoms at the same time.

watch out!

Even if the casualty has already seen a doctor for the same illness, don't delay seeking help again if the condition worsens or new symptoms develop.

Action

1 Call a doctor at once and explain that you suspect meningitis.
2 While waiting, reassure the patient and try to keep him or her cool by bathing with a tepid sponge.
3 If the doctor is delayed or cannot come quickly, call an ambulance.

want to know more?

Viral meningitis is a nasty illness but it is rarely life-threatening. Most people make a full recovery. Bacterial meningitis is more serious. Most cases in the UK are caused by meningococcal bacteria. This bacteria may cause meningitis, or septicaemia, or both. People who get bacterial meningitis usually have symptoms of both meningococcal meningitis and septicaemia (the rash of meningitis is actually a sign of septicaemia). This combination is known as meningococcal disease. For more information about meningitis, contact the Meningitis Research Foundation at www.meningitis.org or via the 24-hour helpline on freefone 080 8800 3344.

Miscarriage

Miscarriage means the loss of a pregnancy before 24 weeks. It can be dangerous if the woman loses a lot of blood. The victim may be very distressed or frightened.

watch out!

Seek urgent medical help even if the bleeding is only slight – it could be a threatened miscarriage, and treatment could prevent loss of the foetus.

Most miscarriages occur within the first 14 weeks of pregnancy, usually due to an abnormality in the foetus. Later miscarriages may be caused by a weak cervix or a severe infection in the mother. Alcohol or drug abuse and smoking all increase the likelihood of a miscarriage. Only one woman in 36 has a repeat miscarriage but the chance of this increases if any of the above risk factors are present. Miscarriage is more common in women under 15 or over 35.

Signs of miscarriage

- ▶ vaginal bleeding in a pregnant woman
- ▶ abdominal pain or cramps
- ▶ symptoms of shock
- ▶ passage of foetus or embryo, or parts of tissue, from vagina

Action

1 Help the woman into a comfortable sitting or lying position and reassure her.
2 Support her back with cushions and bend her knees up over cushions or rolled towels.
3 Offer a pad or clean towel for bleeding.
4 Look for signs of shock and treat if necessary (pages 149-150).
5 Monitor airway, breathing and circulation and be prepared to start resuscitation if necessary (pages 34–41).
6 Collect any material passed from the vagina so that it can be assessed in hospital – but keep it away from the woman's view if possible.

7 Call a doctor at once; if pain or bleeding is severe, call an ambulance.

Other causes of vaginal bleeding

The most usual cause of bleeding from the vagina is menstruation (periods). Bleeding may also indicate:

▶ miscarriage (see above)
▶ recent childbirth (pages 88-89)
▶ recent abortion – if bleeding is severe or accompanied by pain, take or send the victim to hospital
▶ ectopic pregnancy – in which the foetus grows in one of the Fallopian tubes (the tubes connecting the ovaries to the womb) instead of inside the womb. This is highly dangerous if the tube ruptures. There may be severe pain as well as bleeding, and often the victim develops shock. Call an ambulance immediately
▶ sexual assault – ensure that you preserve any evidence, including clothing if the woman wishes to change, and try to discourage the woman from washing until she has been seen by a police doctor
▶ Infection or disease of the vagina, cervix or womb – suggest the woman contacts her own doctor.

did you know?

Approximately one in 100 pregnancies is ectopic.

want to know more?

Help and support
Anyone who has had a miscarriage can contact the Miscarriage Association. Its helpline is open on weekdays from 9am-4pm on 01924 200799; Scottish helpline 0131 334 8883. It has a website at www.miscarriageassociation.org.uk.

Nosebleed

Nosebleeds are common because the blood vessels in the nasal lining are very fragile. The blood vessels may rupture after blowing or sneezing or for no apparent reason.

Recurrent nosebleeds

A person suffering from frequent nosebleeds should see a doctor as this may indicate another more serious condition, such as high blood pressure.

If a child has pushed an object up his or her nose, get the child to a hospital casualty department where medical staff can remove it safely.

Action

1 Ask the casualty to sit down, leaning his head well forwards.

2 Ask the casualty to breathe through his mouth, and not to talk.

3 Put a bowl under his nose and offer a tissue or cloth.

4 Ask the casualty to pinch his nose for 10 minutes. You may have to do this for a young child.

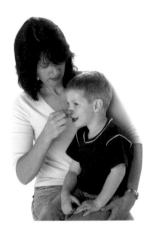

5 Release pressure after 10 minutes. If the nose is still bleeding, pinch again for a further 10 minutes.

6 Once bleeding stops, gently clean the area with lukewarm water.

7 Advise the person to avoid nose-blowing and strenuous physical activity for several hours afterwards.

8 Seek medical help if the bleeding does not stop after 30 minutes.

A watery discharge from the nose may indicate a skull fracture, especially if it follows a head injury. Seek medical attention at once.

Overdose

An overdose is the use of any drug in such an amount that acute adverse physical or mental effects are produced. A drug overdose can happen accidentally, especially in elderly people on multiple medications, who may become confused about their dosages.

Sometimes, a deliberate overdose is an attempt at suicide or a 'cry for help'.

Signs of an overdose

Symptoms will vary depending on what drug has been taken (and how alcohol has interacted with the drug) but may include:

▶ drowsiness, confusion or unconsciousness
▶ agitation, aggression or hallucinations
▶ slurred speech
▶ staggering or loss of balance
▶ slow, shallow breathing
▶ pain in the abdomen or elsewhere
▶ nausea or vomiting

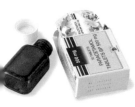

Collect all available packaging used in the overdose as it will help medical staff treat the victim.

Action

1 Check for other danger, such as the gas being left on.
2 Check the casualty's airway and breathing, start resuscitation if necessary (see pages 36–41).
3 Call an ambulance.
4 Find out what has been taken, if you can.
5 Collect any pill bottles or containers to send with the casualty to hospital.
6 Send anything else that may be helpful to medical staff, such as a suicide note or samples of vomit.

Poisoning

Poisons can be swallowed, inhaled, absorbed through the skin or mucous membranes (for example, after splashes in the eye) or injected (for example, drugs, or the venom in a wasp sting).

Signs of poisoning

Symptoms vary depending on the route of entry to the body and the exact substance involved.

Swallowed poisons:

▶ nausea or vomiting

▶ abdominal pain

▶ redness around the mouth

Inhaled poisons:

▶ headache

▶ noisy or difficulty breathing

Any poison:

▶ confusion

▶ altered consciousness or coma

▶ heart and breathing may stop

Once in the body, poisons can be rapidly transported in the bloodstream, and have varying effects.

Many poisons occur naturally, as in poisonous plants, or bacteria and viruses that contaminate food to cause food poisoning. Others, such as household and garden products or industrial chemicals, are manufactured.

Fumes from fires can cause poisoning as well as the effects of smoke inhalation. An overdose of drugs, whether prescribed, brought over the counter or illegal, may cause symptoms of poisoning, as can excess alcohol.

must know

Sources of poisoning

▶ food poisoning causing diarrhoea and/or vomiting – see page 102

▶ drug overdose (swallowed, inhaled or injected) – see page 145

▶ intoxication (drugs or alcohol) – see page 136

▶ gas and fume inhalation – see page 119

▶ skin poisons: chemical burns – see page 84

▶ chemicals in the eye – see page 110

▶ insect stings – see page 76

Action

Seek urgent medical attention for most forms of poisoning.
With a conscious casualty:

1 Ask exactly what was taken and how much.
2 Call an ambulance and give details of the type of poison.
3 If the lips are contaminated, wash with cold water. Give frequent sips of water if there is a chemical burn around the lips (otherwise do not allow the casualty to eat or drink).
4 Monitor airway, breathing and circulation while awaiting the ambulance. Be prepared to start resuscitation if necessary – use a face shield if traces of poison remain around the mouth.
5 Place an unconscious, breathing casualty in the recovery position (see pages 42–43).
6 Send any samples of poison or containers to hospital with the casualty.

watch out!

► do not put yourself in danger if there are toxic chemicals or fumes still around
► never try to induce vomiting if someone has swallowed poison

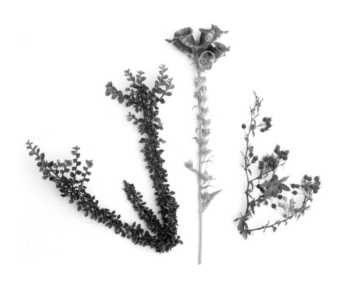

must know

Young children are the most common victims of poisoning in the home.

Bring a sample of the source of poisoning to the hospital with the victim.

Symptoms of poisoning

► drowsiness, confusion or unconsciousness

► agitation, aggression or hallucinations

► staggering or loss of balance

► slow, shallow breathing

► pain in the abdomen or elsewhere

► nausea or vomiting

Swallowed poisons:

► redness around the mouth

Inhaled poisons:

► breathing difficulties

► altered skin colour – blue or bright red

Skin poisons:

► a rash or chemical burn from
  skin contact.

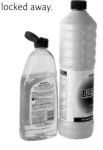

must know

Children are most at risk from poisoning, often from plants or household chemicals. Always keep toxic substances locked away.

Action

1 Check airway and breathing, start resuscitation
  if necessary – use a face shield if traces of poison
  remain around the mouth.

2 Call an ambulance.

3 Send any samples of poison to the hospital, if possible.

Swallowed poisons:

1 Wash the lips and mouth area
  if traces of poison remain.

2 If there is a chemical burn around the lips,
  give frequent sips of water.

Inhaled poisons:

Get the victim to fresh air – drag if necessary.

Skin poisons:

1 Remove any contaminated clothing.

2 Flood the area with running water.

watch out!

► Do not leave casualty alone while awaiting the ambulance.

► Monitor breathing and be prepared to start resuscitation at any time.

► Never try to induce vomiting.

► Do not give any food or drink except to help if the lips are affected by a chemical.

Shock

Shock in a medical sense is quite different from emotional or psychological shock. It means that the body's circulation has failed, and insufficient blood supply is reaching vital organs.

Shock, if progressive, can be life-threatening – eventually the person will become unconscious and the heart and breathing will stop. Shock may be due to any condition that interferes with the normal output of the heart. Blood loss after injury is a common cause. Shock may also be due to the loss of other body fluids in conditions such as burns or protracted vomiting. Other causes of shock include serious injury, heart attack and severe infections. Anaphylactic shock may occur when someone has a very severe allergic reaction (see pages 66–67).

must know

In most cases of physiological shock, reduced blood pressure is a major factor and one of its main features.

Signs of shock
- pale, cold, clammy skin
- weakness and nausea
- dizziness and feeling faint
- rapid, shallow breathing
- grey or blue skin and lips
- gasping for air
- unconsciousness

watch out!

Do not give the casualty anything to eat or drink, in case an anaesthetic is needed to treat whatever is causing the shock.

Action
1 Call an ambulance at once.
2 Treat the cause of shock, for example, severe bleeding or burns (see page 83).
3 Lie the casualty down, preferably on a blanket to give insulation from cold ground. Loosen clothing.

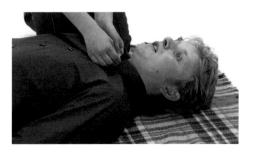

4 Raise the legs by placing them on a chair or cushions to improve blood flow to the heart and brain.

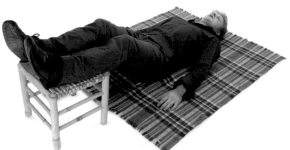

5 Keep the person warm by covering with a blanket or extra clothing, but do not use heat sources such as hot-water bottles.

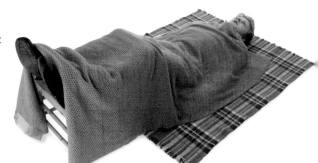

6 Monitor breathing and circulation regularly while awaiting medical help (see pages 34–35). Be prepared to start resuscitation if necessary (see pages 36–41).

7 Place an unconscious but breathing casualty into the recovery position (see pages 42–43).

8 While waiting for the ambulance, treat any other injuries if you can.

must know

Shock can be life-threatening, so always call an ambulance.

Sore throat

A sore throat often accompanies common respiratory infections such as coughs and colds, and may be the first sign that one is developing. It usually gets better on its own or with simple home treatments.

Sore throat symptoms

▶ pain and rawness in the throat

▶ back of the throat may look red and inflamed

▶ pain on swallowing

▶ other cold symptoms: sneezing, runny nose or cough

Action

1 Encourage the person to drink plenty of fluids.

2 Give appropriate painkillers if necessary.

3 Keep the person comfortable in a warm, clean atmosphere.

When to call a doctor

▶ Call a doctor if the sufferer is a young child and develops a high temperature, earache or other worrying symptoms.

▶ See a doctor if the casualty develops a persistent, troublesome cough or if lymph nodes ('glands') around the jaw become swollen and enlarged – he or she may have tonsillitis.

must know

Never give painkillers containing aspirin to a child under 16.

Spinal injury

An injury to the head, neck or back may damage the bones (vertebrae) of the spinal column, the discs between them, the supporting ligaments and muscles, or the spinal cord itself.

Spinal injury can be extremely serious. Damage to the spinal cord or the nerves that run from it may lead to paralysis and other complications, such as an inability to breathe unaided.

Warning signs for spinal injury
- pain and tenderness in the neck or back
- a 'step' in the normally smooth curve of the spine
- weakness or loss of movement or sensation in the legs and sometimes the arms
- abnormal sensation in the limbs – burning, tingling, heaviness or stiffness
- difficulty breathing
- incontinence of urine or faeces

Sometimes such symptoms arise as a result of 'spinal shock', due to injury to the spinal cord that may heal in time. However, if the spinal cord is severed, the damage is likely to be permanent. Any movement of the spinal column that could further damage the spinal cord must therefore be avoided if there is any possibility of spinal injury.

must know
- If you suspect a spinal injury do not move the casualty.
- It the casualty is in the road, put out cones or ask someone to divert any traffic.

Likely causes of spinal injury
- fall from a height
- fall or impact onto the head (such as when diving into a shallow swimming pool)
- falling off a horse or motorcycle
- an injury from a collapsed rugby scrum

- fall that twists or bends the neck, for example landing awkwardly on a trampoline, or while doing gymnastics
- a heavy object falling on the head, neck or back
- a road accident, especially a head-on collision

Action

1 Send someone to call an ambulance immediately, and to tell the controller that you suspect a spinal injury.
2 Tell a conscious casualty not to move.
3 Kneel behind the casualty's head and place your hands on either side of the head to hold it still. Keep the head, neck and spine in line. Do not allow the head or neck to move, and do not move your hands until the ambulance arrives. Rest your arms on your knees to prevent fatigue.

watch out!

Remember that a spinal injury may be associated with head injury (see page 124), which can also be serious.

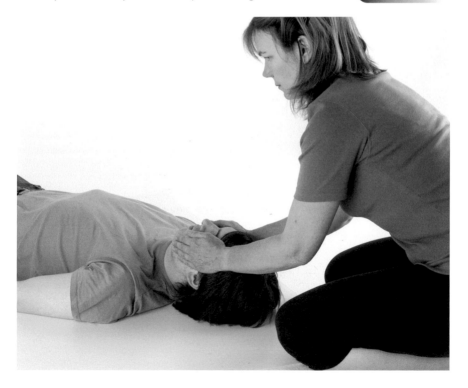

4 If there is anyone else around, ask for help. Tell the person to fetch some padding, such as rolled towels or firm cushions, and place it around the casualty's neck and shoulders (with your hands still in place).

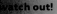
5 For an unconscious casualty, use the jaw-thrust method to open the airway (see must know box). Do not put the person into the recovery position (see pages 42–43) unless you are alone and it is absolutely necessary that you leave to fetch help.

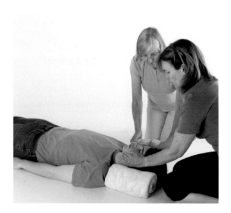

6 Monitor breathing and circulation and be prepared to start resuscitation if necessary (page 34–41), using the jaw-thrust method to keep the airway open. If you have a helper, one of you should hold the head steady while the other performs resuscitation.

must know

The jaw-thrust method
This is an alternative method of opening the airway and checking breathing. It should be used for any casualty with a possible spinal injury, as it avoids tilting the head.
Kneel down and place your hands on either side of the victim's face, placing your fingertips at the angle of the jaw on each side. Gently lift the jaw to open the airway.

Splinters

Splinters are very common and may be slivers of wood, metal, glass or other objects. The wound itself is rarely serious but there is a risk of infection.

It is usually easy to tell when you have a splinter. There is pain and a sliver of material protruding from a tiny wound. There may be a pinprick mark on the skin.

must know

If the splinter is so embedded that you cannot grasp it, or if you cannot get it out or it breaks off, seek medical attention.

Action

1 Sit or lie the casualty down with the area affected resting on a flat surface.

2 Take a pair of metal tweezers and sterilise the ends by holding over a flame until they glow red. Allow the ends to cool.

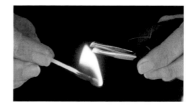

3 Firmly grasp the end of the splinter and pull along the line in which it went in.

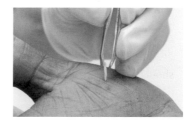

4 Squeeze the wound slightly to flush a little blood out, then clean with soap and water or an antiseptic solution or spray.

5 Cover with a dry sterile dressing.

watch out!

Ask if the victim has had full immunisation against tetanus, and advise them to see a doctor if not.

Sprains and strains

Sudden wrenching or twisting forces can lead to overstretching or tearing of muscles (strains) or of the ligaments and tendons around a joint (sprains).

A sprain or strain is indicated by a sudden pain and tenderness around a joint accompanied by difficulty in moving it. There may be localised swelling, cramping or bruising in the affected area. Sometimes a muscle or tendon is completely ruptured. Often the result of sporting activities, these soft-tissue injuries are sometimes hard to distinguish from fractures.

Action

Initial treatment is to follow the RICE procedure:

1 Rest – stop using the injured part. Ask the casualty to sit or lie down and rest the injured part on something soft, such as a cushion or pillow.

2 Ice – apply an ice pack or cold compress (see page 50) to reduce bruising and swelling. If an ice pack is unavailable, a packet of frozen peas or similar wrapped in a towel makes an excellent substitute.

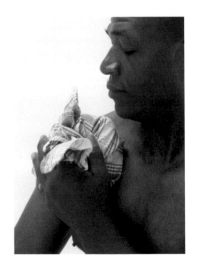

must know

Where to look

▶ the wrist and ankle are the most common sites of sprains

▶ muscle tears may occur in the calf, thigh, neck or lower back

3 Compression – apply gentle pressure with some soft padding secured with a bandage. This reduces swelling and bruising.

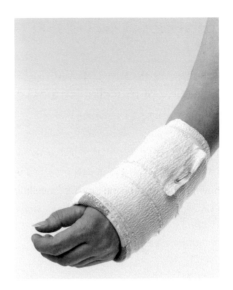

A clean towel or piece of cloth can be used as padding when making a compression bandage.

4 Elevation – if possible, raise and support the affected part to reduce blood flow and minimise bruising. For example, ask the casualty to rest the injured area on a cushion on top of a stool.
If the injury is to the lower back, advise the casualty to lie down on a firm surface.

When to see a doctor

▶ If the casualty has severe pain, is unable to bear weight on or use the injured limb, take or send him to hospital – there could be a fracture and an X-ray may be necessary.

▶ Seek prompt medical advice if symptoms have not improved after several hours despite RICE treatment.

Stitch and cramp

Both a stitch and cramp are painful muscular spasms, often caused by exercise, though cramp may also occur spontaneously especially at night.

A stitch is a sudden, sharp pain in a muscle, usually on one side of the chest or abdomen. Cramp is the sudden painful spasm of a muscle, often in the calf or foot and sometimes occuring at night.

Stitches and cramps commonly occur after an intense bout of exercise, due to waste products accumulating too fast for the body to disperse them. Cramp can also be the result of a disturbance in the body's salt and water balance, such as from profuse sweating.

watch out!

Cramp while swimming can be dangerous – build up a training routine slowly.

Action

1 Ask the person to sit quietly and rest; the pain of a stitch should pass quickly.

2 Cramp will pass by itself, but you can help by stretching and massaging the affected area until it subsides.

3 If severe pain persists for more than a few minutes, the cause may be something else and the casualty needs medical attention.

4 For night cramps, see your doctor who may be able to prescribe drugs to relieve the problem.

watch out!

See a doctor if you suffer repeated cramps as they may be caused by an underlying disorder.

Strangulation

Strangulation occurs when someone's airway and the blood flow to the brain are cut off by pressure on the neck or throat. If breathing and circulation are not restored very quickly, brain damage or death may follow.

Signs of strangulation

▶ noose or constriction around the neck
▶ breathing laboured or absent
▶ unconsciousness
▶ grey skin and blue lips
▶ congestion of face with prominent veins

Action

1 Ask someone to call an ambulance immediately.
2 Handle the head very carefully after hanging (see pages 152-154).
3 Support the casualty to take the weight from the neck.

4 Cut through the constriction – do not waste time trying to untie knots.
5 If using a knife, cut very carefully away from the victim's neck.
6 If the casualty is unconscious, check breathing and circulation and perform resuscitation if necessary (pages 34-41).
7 Place an unconscious casualty who is breathing in the recovery position (see pages 42-43).

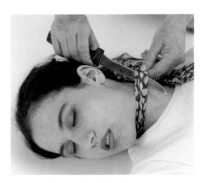

Cut away from the victim's neck

Stroke

A stroke is caused by a loss of blood supply and damage to a part of the brain as a result of an artery becoming blocked with a blood clot or, sometimes, bursting and bleeding into the brain. Early treatment can prevent long-term loss of function.

Symptoms of stroke

These vary according to the part of the brain affected, and may include:

▶ weakness or paralysis down one side of the body

▶ loss of speech or slurred speech

▶ dribbling

▶ confusion; the victim may appear drunk

▶ sudden, severe 'thunderclap' headache

▶ involuntary urination or bowel movement

▶ loss of consciousness

watch out!

Do not give the victim anything to eat or drink in case swallowing is impaired.

Action

1 Call an ambulance.

2 Monitor breathing and circulation (see pages 34–35). Be prepared to start resuscitation if necessary (see pages 36–41).

3 Make the victim comfortable; mop up any dribble with a towel.

4 Reassure the victim but avoid too much conversation if he or she is having difficulty speaking.

want to know more?

For more information about strokes, contact the Stroke Association via its website (www.stroke.org.uk) or phone 0845 3033 100.

Suffocation

Suffocation occurs when insufficient oxygen reaches the lungs. The medical term is asphyxia. Anyone who has nearly suffocated should be checked by a doctor afterwards.

Suffocation may be due to obstruction or damage to the airways, as in strangulation (see page 159), choking (see pages 90-93), drowning (pages 104-105), smothering, or crush injuries (see page 97) affecting the chest and impairing breathing. It can also occur when someone is trapped in a confined space with no air supply, or during gas or smoke inhalation (see page 119).

must know

Suffocation is one of the most common causes of accidental death in babies and children under 14.

Signs of suffocation
▶ difficulty breathing and speaking
▶ grey-blue skin, lips and nails
▶ flaring of the nostrils
▶ impaired consciousness

Action
1 Call an ambulance immediately.
2 If the cause is fume or smoke inhalation, get the victim out into fresh air if possible.
3 Open the airway and remove any obvious obstruction to breathing (see pages 34-35) .
4 Check breathing and circulation and start resuscitation if necessary (see pages 34-41).
5 Place an unconscious but breathing casualty in the recovery position (pages 42-43) while awaiting help.

watch out!

Do not place yourself in danger by entering a space filled with smoke or toxic fumes – call for help.

Sunburn

Sunburn is the inflammation and reddening of the skin caused by overexposure to ultraviolet radiation. This can happen after lying in the sun or using a sunbed.

Signs of sunburn
- red, sore skin
- later on, peeling or even blistering skin

Action

1 Get the casualty into the shade, preferably indoors, or cover with light clothing or a towel.

2 Cool the skin with tepid water – a sponge or a bath – for 10 minutes.

3 Give plenty of sips of cool water to drink.

4 Use a cooling after-sun lotion on the skin.

5 Check for associated heat stroke and treat accordingly (see pages 128–129).

must know

Sunburn should be avoided, by covering up or using protective suncreams, because of its link with skin cancer.

watch out!

Sunburn can develop in as little as 20 minutes. Play it safe in the sun.

When to see a doctor
- if the area burned is extensive or the burn is severe, especially if blisters develop
- if a baby or small child gets sunburned
- a sunburn victim develops a headache, raised temperature or confusion

Toothache and detached tooth

Toothache is usually due to dental decay. A tooth that has been knocked out may be saved if you can re-implant it, or preserve it while seeking urgent dental care.

Toothache

Action:

1 Use mild painkillers or a hot-water bottle wrapped in a towel and held against the cheek to ease toothache.
2 Clove oil applied to the gum area may also relieve pain.
3 Advise the casualty to see her dentist urgently.

Knocked-out tooth

Action:

1 Hold the tooth firmly and gently push it back into the socket.
2 Wrap a gauze pad around the tooth and ask the casualty to grip firmly between the upper and lower teeth.
3 If you cannot re-implant the tooth, place it in milk or water, or have the victim hold it in their cheek to prevent it from drying out.
4 Seek urgent dental advice.

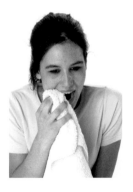

Wounds

When treating open wounds it is important to protect both yourself and the casualty from any risk of infection. The most likely source of contamination is body fluids – saliva, vomit or other secretions and, especially, blood.

Hygiene first

Aim to avoid 'cross contamination'. You need to protect yourself from any infection carried by the casualty, and to protect the casualty from your germs and from any germs or dirt at the scene that could be on your hands. Whenever possible, before touching a casualty you should:

▶ wash your hands thoroughly, or use an antiseptic solution or spray

▶ cover any cuts or grazes of your own with plasters

▶ put on a pair of disposable gloves. If no gloves are available, clean plastic bags will substitute or, where appropriate, ask the casualty to handle his or her own wound and dressings.

Types of wound

Grazes

In these superficial skin abrasions, the surface layer of skin is scraped off. The main first aid problem is the removal of embedded small particles, such as gravel or grit.

Incised wounds

These are clean cuts, as from a razor blade or knife. They may bleed profusely, and deep wounds may damage underlying tendons, nerves or blood vessels.

watch out!

If you do accidentally become contaminated with a casualty's blood or secretions, wash the area thoroughly with soap or an antiseptic solution and seek medical advice afterwards.

Lacerations

Crushing or ripping forces may produce tears in the skin and there is often damage to underlying tissues, and a high risk of infection.

Puncture or stab wounds

Although these may leave only a small entry wound, they carry a high risk of infection due to their depth. Stab wounds to the trunk may cause life-threatening damage to internal organs.

Bullet wounds

The point of entry of a bullet usually leaves a small, neat hole. Underlying damage may be extremely serious. If the bullet passes right through the body the exit wound will be large and messy.

Treating wounds

See bandaging techniques (pages 52–59). Provided there is no embedded object, apply direct pressure or a bandage with padding to stem the bleeding.

1 Clean the wound with soap and water or antiseptic. Use cotton wool or gauze pads and use each one once only. Wipe from the wound outwards, to avoid contamination with bacteria from surrounding skin.

2 If any particles in the wound do not come out with gentle washing, do not attempt to remove them.

3 Apply a sterile dressing large enough to overlap the wound edges on all sides and, if necessary, put a bandage on top to hold it in place.

4 If blood seeps through the dressing, apply a second one on top.

5 Check that any bandage is not impairing circulation (see page 59).

6 With severe bleeding, call an ambulance and watch for signs of shock (see pages 149–150).

Seek medical attention for:

► face wounds (possible scarring)

► cuts to the hands or feet (possible nerve or tendon damage)

► particles or embedded objects left in the wound

► deep or heavily contaminated wounds – the casualty may need a tetanus shot

Call an ambulance if there is:

► severe bleeding

► signs of shock

► any penetrating wound to the trunk

► any stab or bullet wound

watch out!

Never attempt to remove an object embedded in a wound, as this could increase damage to underlying tissues.

Embedded object

If there is an object in the wound, you need to stem bleeding without pressing directly on the object.

1 Apply firm pressure to either side of the object, pressing inwards towards it.

2 Carefully place soft padding around the object, if possible up to the level of the object.

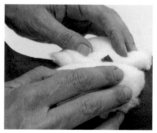

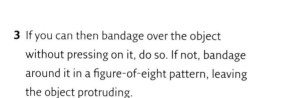

3 If you can then bandage over the object without pressing on it, do so. If not, bandage around it in a figure-of-eight pattern, leaving the object protruding.

4 Take or send the victim to hospital.

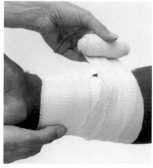

Amputation

Sometimes fingers or toes, or even larger limbs, are severed in an accident. Modern surgical techniques often enable the part to be reattached, provided that it is kept in good condition before and during transport to hospital.

1 Lie the casualty down, control bleeding at the stump and apply a clean dressing or bandage.

2 Treat shock if necessary (see pages 149–150).

3 Retrieve the severed part and place in a thick layer of gauze or fabric padding, or place in a plastic bag which you then blow into and tie to create an air cushion around the part.

4 Place this in another bag or a rigid container of ice cubes or crushed ice (frozen peas will substitute).

5 Label the container with the victim's name and the time of amputation and give it to the ambulance crew.

watch out!

► Do not wash the severed part.
► Do not allow the part to come into direct contact with ice.
► Do not allow the casualty to eat or drink, as he or she will need an anaesthetic.

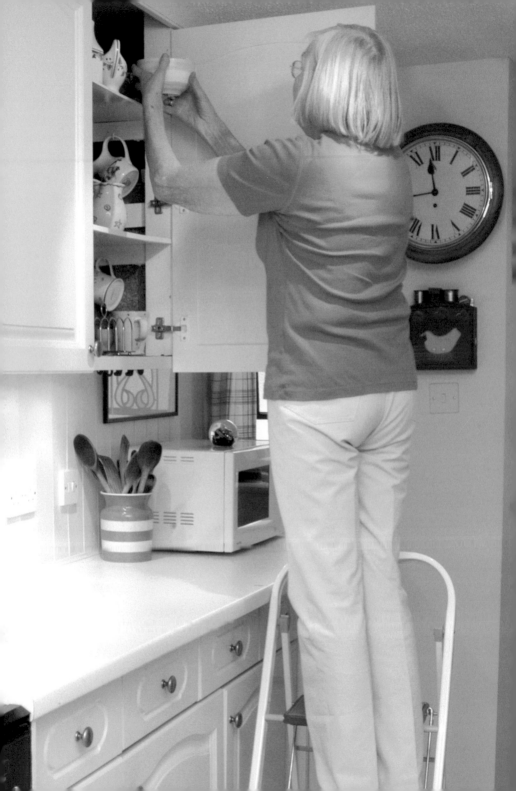

4 Accident prevention

Knowing what to do at the scene of an accident is invaluable, but there is much you can do to avoid such a situation occuring in the first instance. This section looks at how you can be aware of potential dangers while at home and out and about. Many of the key hazards you may face were detailed in the first section of this book. The following pages describe the precautions and measures you should take to modify your environment and make it a safe place for yourself and your family.

Accident prevention at home

More accidents occur in the home than anywhere else. Everyone should be aware of potential dangers and how they can be avoided.

Safety in the kitchen

Some of the most serious accidents happen in the kitchen and food preparation areas. Always make sure that children are fully supervised in the kitchen.

Cooking

Many fires and scalding accidents occur through the misuse of equipment. Make sure that you read the safety instructions that accompany any new kitchen appliance before using.

▶ never leave hot pans unattended – especially frying or chip pans
▶ turn pan handles inwards
▶ use the back rings on a hob whenever possible
▶ do not cook on a gas hob with flowing sleeves, loose clothing or loose hair
▶ don't allow fat or grease to build up on cookers and hobs
▶ never fill a pan more than one-third full of oil
▶ don't put wet food into hot oil
▶ never throw water on a frying-pan or chip-pan fire – use a fire blanket or fire extinguisher, or smother with a wrung-out damp towel; do not move the pan for at least 30 minutes afterwards
▶ a thermostat-controlled deep fat fryer is safer than a chip pan

Worktop safety

Plan worktop and storage areas carefully.
A well-organised kitchen will reduce the number of potential hazards.

▶ don't reach above a boiling kettle
▶ avoid hanging curtains near the hob, oven or toaster, and don't leave flammable items such as tea towels, oven gloves or kitchen rolls nearby

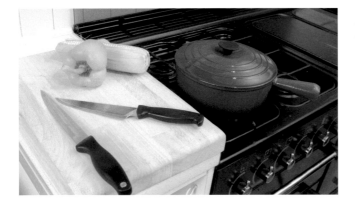

Keep pan handles turned in and away from where children might be able to reach them. Sharp knives should also be kept out of reach.

▶ make sure you keep electric cables from trailing near the hob
▶ clean crumbs out of the toaster regularly
▶ keep a clear surface next to the oven for hot dishes

Sharp edges

Sharp or serrated edges are a constant hazard in kitchen areas.
These tips will help you to work more safely.
▶ never load sharp knives in a dishwasher
  with the point upwards
▶ keep knives on a magnetic knife rack fixed to the wall,
  or in a drawer or a divided tray. They should all point
  in the same direction. Never fumble in a knife drawer
  without looking
▶ don't leave cans with sharp edges lying around – rinse,
  put the lid inside and place in a recycling box immediately

---

must know

Safety in the kitchen
▶ Keep a fire blanket or fire extinguisher clearly visible
  and properly maintained.
▶ Ensure that all floor coverings are non-slip and keep
  the floor clean and dry – mop up any spills at once.
▶ Don't cook if you are tired, have had too much alcohol
  or have taken medicines that may make you drowsy.

Reducing the risk of food poisoning

It can never be repeated enough that people working where food is being prepared should always wash their hands before preparing food and after using the lavatory. Here are some other measures to prevent food poisoning:

▶ cover any cuts on your hands with adhesive dressings before food preparation
▶ don't cough or sneeze near food
▶ keep pets well away from food-preparation areas and wash pet dishes separately
▶ don't keep food warm; re-heated foods should be 'piping hot' and served immediately
▶ keep uncooked meat and poultry on the bottom shelf of the fridge, where it cannot drip onto other foods
▶ use separate chopping boards for raw meats and poultry
▶ avoid food that is past its 'use by' date
▶ store food in covered containers in the fridge

Precautions in the bathroom

There are several ways to make the bathroom a safer place. The following are practical ideas for avoiding accidents:

▶ use non-slip mats in bath and shower and a non-slip bathmat on the floor
▶ never leave a baby or young child alone in the bath
▶ apply plastic safety film to glass shower doors and cubicles to keep glass in place if it breaks
▶ never mix cleaning fluids and bleach – this can cause poisonous fumes
▶ keep all tablets and medicines in a locked cabinet
▶ never use electrical items (other than a shaver in an approved socket) in a bathroom, even if it's plugged in elsewhere
▶ don't change light bulbs straight after someone has had a bath or shower – wait until any steam or condensation has cleared; ensure your hands are scrupulously dry

must know

If you have children, elderly or frail household members, hot tap water should be no hotter than 46°C. Fit a thermostatic mixing valve if possible (you need a plumber or builder for this). Otherwise, turn down the temperature setting on the hot-water tank.

Older people

Serious accidents involving older people usually happen in the kitchen or on the stairs and result in arm, leg and shoulder injuries. Those over 75 are most at risk and suffer the most severe injuries. Accidents involving older people tend to be due to frailty and failing health.

Regular eye check-ups are important for safety in the home. Injuries due to overbalancing can be prevented by checking with your doctor whether any of the medications you take cause dizziness as a side effect. If you feel your balance is impaired in any way, talk to your doctor.

Preventing falls

There are several ways to minimise the likelihood of falls and fractures:
- keep halls and stairs well lit
- fix any loose or worn stair carpet
- fit non-slip pads under rugs
- keep main routes through rooms clear: avoid leaving clutter on the floor
- have a sturdy handrail on stairs; fit handrails in corridors if necessary
- put non-slip mats in front of kitchen and bathroom sinks, and baths and showers
- don't climb on chairs to do high level jobs: use a proper stool, steps or platform
- if you have to use a ladder, position it securely and have someone brace the base while you climb

Electricity and fire

Electricity, fire and heat can cause some of the most serious injuries in and around the home. Fires can start very suddenly and spread quickly through a household.

Electricity

Always check and follow safety instructions for all appliances. If you have any doubt about a piece of equipment, stop using it and have it checked by a qualified contractor. Here are some useful tips to keep your home safe:

▶ don't overload sockets or adaptors
▶ avoid having trailing wires
▶ unplug televisions at night and during storms
▶ keep electrical equipment and cables away from water; do not touch appliances or switches with wet hands
▶ don't put anything damp or liquid (like wet clothes or vases of flowers) near an electrical appliance
▶ beware of worn flexes or frayed leads – replace appliance or have it repaired
▶ always use the correct fuses in plugs; have loose electric sockets replaced
▶ never use a bulb with a higher wattage than is recommended for the lamp, its shade or the light fitting
▶ keep ventilation slots in electronic equipment clear, and don't let any liquid drip or splash into them
▶ fit a Residual Current Device (RCD) to bathroom and kitchen circuits

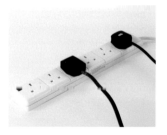

The sensible use of an adaptor will avoid overloading a plug socket.

Home safety: Fire!

Lives are always in danger when a fire starts but there are many simple ways in which you can prevent them from happening in the first place:

▸ keep lighters, matches and flammable materials away from children and heat sources

▸ always use a fireguard

▸ never dry or air clothes on a fireguard or near a fire or heater

▸ keep curtains and soft furnishings away from cooking equipment, heaters or open fires

▸ never leave candles burning near a curtain or other flammable material, or where they could be knocked over; use flame-proof candle holders; always snuff out candles when you leave the room

▸ never drape fabric over a bulb or lamp

▸ never put a cigarette down except in an ashtray. Don't leave cigarettes burning in ashtrays: stub them out and throw away in a suitable container outside, or dunk in water – especially last thing at night

▸ don't smoke in bed

▸ check electric blankets are undamaged before using in the winter and don't go to sleep with the blanket switched on

▸ don't leave a hair-dryer switched on if you are not using it

▸ replace old soft furnishings containing foam

Smoke alarms

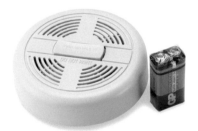

Fit proper smoke alarms – at least one per floor. Alarms should be attached to the ceiling. Test alarms **at least once a week**. Change the batteries at least annually.

If there is a fire that you cannot contain, get everyone out of the building immediately – call for help from a neighbouring house or mobile phone. Never delay or go back for possessions or pets.

If you have to climb out of a window to escape a fire, don't jump – lower yourself out, hanging onto the ledge, so you have less distance to fall.

Child safety

Children most at risk of a home accident are within the 0-4 age group. Most injuries can be prevented through a greater awareness of dangers in the home environment.

Keep hazards out of reach

It is impossible to cater for every likely scenario at home but the following specific advice for keeping children safe may help. Children should be supervised at all times.

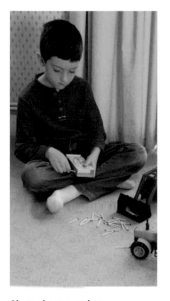

Always keep matches in a safe place out of the reach of inquisitive children.

Children will always be inquisitive and, as a result, in danger of accidents. Avoid putting tempting objects above a fireplace, and keep the following items out of children's reach:

▶ hot liquids – don't carry a child and a hot drink at the same time
▶ medicines and household chemicals – keep them in childproof containers
▶ cigarettes, lighters, matches and flammable items
▶ plastic bags
▶ sharp implements – scissors, sewing materials, razors and nail files
▶ personal care items – perfume, aftershave, hair dyes and hairspray.

must know

Fire safety
▶ Plan fire escape routes – especially from bedrooms.
▶ Practise fire drills with older children.

Toys and equipment

All toys and equipment must meet safety standards. Always check the label to make sure that the toy is suitable for the age group of the child. Do not let young children play with any toys that contain small parts as there is a risk of choking.

▶ do not use 'sit-in' baby walkers
▶ always use a safety harness in a high chair
▶ all spaces between bars – banisters, cot bars, railings etc – should be less than 6cm (2.5 inches) across – about the width of a soft-drinks can
▶ any toy box large enough for a child to climb into should have a lightweight lid with holes in it

A safe home

There are many very simple and effective ways to keep your child safe at home:

▶ fit approved locks or child-safety catches even on downstairs windows
▶ fit cupboard locks or safety catches to all kitchen cupboards and drawers, especially those containing knives, heavy pans, fragile items, alcohol, small food items (such as dried pasta, peas or beans) and cleaning materials
▶ fit stairgates at the top and bottom of stairs
▶ fit an approved fireguard, screwed to the wall, over any working fireplace (this is a **legal requirement** with a child in the house)
▶ plug all unused electric sockets with safety covers
▶ fix corner guards to sharp edges of furniture
▶ screw heavy furniture – like bookcases and shelf units – securely to the wall with metal brackets
▶ keep children off wet tiled floors
▶ keep doors on washing machines, dishwashers and tumble dryers closed

Sleeping safely

▶ place babies on their backs to sleep
▶ avoid pillows, duvets or blankets for babies – use sheets and cellular blankets only
▶ don't put stuffed animals or soft toys into a baby's cot
▶ ensure that nightwear is non-flammable
▶ avoid bunk beds for children under the age of six

Preventing children from choking

Children can inhale and choke on bits of food. They can also swallow small items found around the house. Toys should be appropriate for the age of the child. If in doubt, you can buy a 'choke tester' (very inexpensive) for assessing the diameter of small objects; don't give your child anything that fails the test.

Remember that some toys have small parts that are not meant to come off – but do. Test the eyes on dolls and teddies. Here are some other child-prevention tactics:

► supervise children playing with balloons – a fragment of rubber from a burst balloon could choke a child
► among the most dangerous choking hazards are marbles, buttons, coins, beads, button batteries, small pieces of crayon, erasers and small stones or bits of gravel
► always supervise meals, especially for children under four, and don't rush their eating
► make sure they chew properly if eating nuts, seeds, popcorn, grapes, chunks of meat or hard vegetables like raw carrots
► don't let children move around or lie down while eating

Children and water

Children should always be supervised when in or near water. Even very shallow areas such as a pond or paddling pool present a very real danger of drowning.

► never, ever leave babies or small children alone with water, even for a few seconds; if the phone or doorbell goes at bathtime and you must answer, take your dripping baby or toddler with you
► always test water temperature before putting a child in a bath – it should feel cooler than an adult bath
► supervise children in paddling pools at all times; after use, drain the pool and turn upside-down so it cannot collect rainwater

- cover water butts with netting
- securely fence all pools and ponds; be wary of other people's gardens
- always insist that children wear a lifejacket of the right size when on open stretches of water
- teach children to swim, and warn them never to swim alone

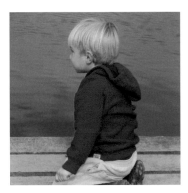

Avoiding poisoning

Most poisoning incidents involve household products such as bleach or cosmetics. Make sure that anything that could cause harm is kept out of reach or locked away. Call an ambulance if you think your child may have swallowed a dangerous substance.

Don't leave children unattended near water.

- fit a carbon-monoxide detector and have cooking and heating appliances serviced and flues checked regularly for poisonous gas emissions
- keep all household chemicals in a high or locked cupboard
- keep all drugs and medicines in a high-level, locked medicine cabinet
- never put dangerous chemicals into old food containers or bottles
- don't leave tablets or medicines on bedside tables or bathroom shelves – lock them away
- warn grandparents to be careful with their medications – and watch Grandma's handbag in case of prying toddler fingers
- explain to children the dangers of eating berries and remove poisonous plants from your garden (see also page 182)
- keep sheds securely locked; even so, put poisonous chemicals such as pesticides, weedkiller or slug pellets on a high shelf out of reach

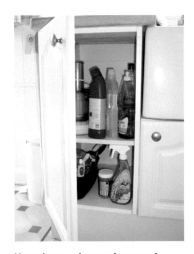

Never leave poisonous items such as bleach or other cleaning products within children's reach.

Out and about

Accidents can happen in the most unlikely situations, but there are many steps you can take to protect yourself and your loved ones when you go out.

Out and about with children

Road sense has to be drummed into children – you can never repeat road safety messages too often. When visiting friends and relatives, check their houses and gardens for hazards before letting children roam freely.

Road safety

▶ don't push a pushchair or buggy ahead
   of you into the road when waiting to cross
▶ don't let young children play in the street
▶ teach children road safety rules from an early age – but
   don't let them cross a road unsupervised until age eight
▶ don't let a child under 10 cycle on the road without an adult
▶ all children should have proper training before cycling
   on the road unaccompanied
▶ ensure that children always wear an approved helmet when riding a bike,
   scooter, skateboard or roller blades; properly fitted helmets reduce the
   risk of head injury and brain damage by up to 88 per cent

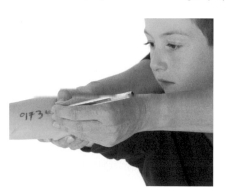

A phone number written on his arm will help to reunite a lost child with his parents.

Must know

Bike helmets
A bike helmet should be worn flat on top of the head – not tilted back at an angle.
The chin strap should be tight.

New places

- in crowded public places or at large gatherings, write your mobile phone number on your child's arm, and switch your mobile on so you can be contacted

Car safety

Some car-safety rules apply to passengers; others to drivers. All are designed to get you to your destination safely and in comfort:

- buy new, age-appropriate car seats and ensure that they are properly fitted: rear-facing seats are safer for babies up to 13kg (29lbs)
- always check where your children are before reversing out of the garage or drive
- don't let a child use electric car windows
- teach your child always to exit the car on the pavement side
- never put a child under 12 in the front seat of a car, or drive with a child on a parent's lap
- always ensure passenger seat belts are securely fastened. Never 'double up' with two children in one belt.

Be a safe driver

- have the car serviced regularly and check car brakes, lights, oil and water before long journeys
- never drink and drive
- don't use a mobile phone, even with a hands-free kit, while driving
- don't drive when overtired: if you feel sleepy, pull over immediately, have a brief nap or get some fresh air and walk around for a while
- carry a first aid kit and emergency items (see pages 10–11)

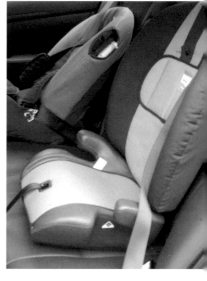

Fit car seats suitable for each child's age and bodyweight in the back of the car.

In the garden

Gardens can provide a source of relaxation for stressed adults or adventure parks for toddlers. However you choose to use your garden, it's best to make it safe.

Safety in the garden

Gardens can present an obstacle course to the very young as well as to the frail or elderly. To minimise the risk of accidents, it's a good idea to:

▶ deal with tripping hazards such as piles of rubble, uneven paving stones or unwound hose pipes

▶ watch out for slipping hazards, such as puddles of water on paving slabs, or moss on steps or pavements

▶ make sure gates and fences are secure if children use the garden

▶ be careful with ladders – whether pruning or cleaning out gutters – always position securely and try to get a helper to support the ladder

Play areas

▶ don't use pesticides or weed killers on or near vegetables you intend to eat, or near any children's play areas

▶ if you have children living with you or visiting, check garden plants and remove any that are poisonous, such as deadly nightshade, laburnum or foxglove

▶ trim back prickly or thorny plants from areas where people walk or children play

▶ don't put rubbish bins that could attract wasps near eating or play areas

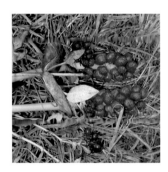

Warn children of the dangers of eating plants, especially berries.

- check children's play equipment and garden furniture before each summer to make sure that it is still stable and intact; discard any broken, rotten or rusty items
- place children's play equipment on a soft surface – such as lawn, sand or special protective coatings

Garden tools
- don't leave tools lying around
- don't mow the lawn while children are playing nearby
- don't refuel a petrol lawnmower when it is hot; never fill the tank completely, to allow for expansion in heated oil
- store petrol only in an approved metal or plastic container designed for the purpose in a locked, ventilated shed

Electrical equipment
- if you have an electric lawnmower, hedge trimmer or similar equipment, instal a residual current device (RCD) on the socket outlet, to cut the power if you accidentally slice through the cable; test it every three months
- never use electrical gardening tools when they are wet
- never adjust or remove items stuck in lawnmower blades without disconnecting the power of an electric mower or removing the wire from the spark plug in a petrol one

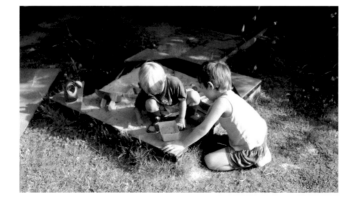

Do not allow pets into children's sandpits or other play areas. Check that these areas are clean before children play in them.

Useful organisations

The following organisations will provide information on first aid, how to become a trained first aider and general advice on keeping safe at home and out and about.

British Red Cross

The British Red Cross trains more than 150,000 people in first aid every year, preparing them to cope with emergencies both at home and at work. It runs first aid courses for all ages.
For further information contact:
- British Red Cross UK Office
  44 Moorfields
  London EC2Y 9AL
  Telephone: 0870 170 7000
  www.redcross.org.uk

St John Ambulance

Provides first aid and medical support services, caring services in support of community needs and education, training and personal development to young people. It runs first aid courses for the public, for schools, and in the workplace.
For further information contact:
- St John Ambulance
  27 St. John's Lane
  London EC1M 4BU
  Tel: 08700 10 49 50
  www.sja.org.uk

BBC First Aid Action

An online course designed to help the general public understand the fundamental aspects of first aid.
The site enables users to receive a certificate by successfully completing a training course with a recognised first aid organisation. It provides links to local first aid courses. For further information see:
- www.bbc.co.uk/health/
  first_aid_action

Royal Society for the Prevention of Accidents

RoSPA is a registered charity campaigning and offering information and training on safety issues. It is involved in safety promotion and prevention of accidents in all areas of life – at work, in the home, and on the roads, in schools, at leisure and on (or near) water.
- RoSPA House,
  Edgbaston Park
  353 Bristol Road
  Birmingham B5 7ST
  Tel: 0121 248 2000
  www.rospa.com

Addaction

This is an organisation that helps individuals and communities manage the effects of drug and alcohol misuse by providing effective services.

Addaction's website provides links to find out how to recognise drug misuse and what you can do help someone. For further information see:

▶ www.addaction.org.uk

FRANK

FRANK is a drugs awareness campaign aimed at young people and parents who need help with a drug or alcohol problem.

The website and telephone line provides free confidential drugs information and advice 24 hours a day. For further information:

▶ a helpline 0800 77 66 00 is available for anyone who needs help
▶ website talktofrank.com offers interactive help. Email frank@talktofrank.com
▶ textphone is available on 0800 917 8765

Health and Safety Executive

The HSE is the national organisation responsible for health and safety regulations. This includes:

▶ reviewing and maintaining approved codes of practice, and guidance and providing advice as requested;
▶ enforcing safety at work regulations

The Health and Safety Executive is also the government organisation that approves and monitors providers of *First Aid at Work* training courses. It offers information on legal requirements for *First Aid at Work* certification in employment, and its website contains links to specialist areas such as offshore employment.

All public enquiries relating to occupational health and safety should in the first instance be directed to HSE. For further information:

▶ HSE Infoline: 0845 345 0055
▶ online information on first aid training can be found at: www.hse.gov.uk/firstaid/index.htm

NHS Direct

NHS Direct is a 24-hour nurse advice and health information service, providing confidential information on:

▶ health conditions
▶ local healthcare services
▶ self help and support

For further information:

▶ call 0845 46 47 (local rate)
▶ visit www.nhsdirect.nhs.uk
▶ in Scotland NHS24 can be contacted on 08454 24 24 24

Index

Entries in the A-Z of first aid treatments are listed in bold.

Acknowledgements

Need to know? First Aid was produced for HarperCollins by Book Creation Illustrated Ltd, Mitre House, 44-46 Fleet Street, London EC4Y 1BN (email: info@bookcreation.com):

For Book Creation Illustrated:

Managing Editor	David Popey
Art Editor	Keith Miller
Project Editor	Helen Spence
Proofreader	Kim Davies
Indexer	Marie Lorimer
Publishing Director	Hal Robinson

Author:	Sheena Meredith MB BS MRCS (Eng) LRCP (Lond)
Consultant:	Dr Vincent Forte BA MB BS MRCGP MSc DA

With many thanks to:
Roddy Paine Photographic Studio, and to Dr Rodger Charlton for his helpful guidance in reviewing this book.

Picture credits:
LifeART: 88 and 89
Dr P. Marazzi/Science Photo Library: 65
Cordelia Molloy/Science Photo Library: 44
Paul Rapson/Science Photo Library: 67
Caroline Martin: 69, 77, 83
Helen Spence: 19, 21, 24, 179, 182, 183
Paul Whitehill/Science Photo Library: 140

☼ Collins need to know?

Look out for these recent titles in Collins' practical and accessible need to know? series.

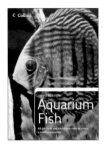 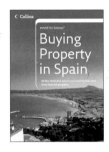 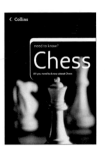 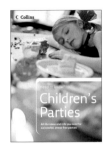

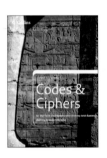 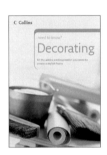 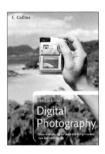 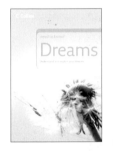

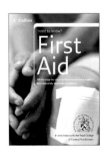 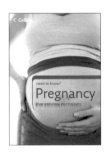 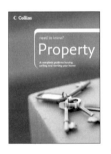 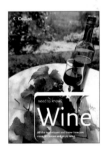

Other titles in the series:

Antique Marks
Birdwatching
Body Language
Buying Property in France
Card Games
DIY
Dog Training
Drawing & Sketching
Golf
Guitar

How to Lose Weight
Kama Sutra
Kings and Queens
Knots
Low GI/GL Diet
Pilates
Poker
Speak French
Speak Italian
Speak Spanish

Stargazing
Watercolour
Weddings
Woodworking
The World
Yoga
Zodiac Types

**To order any of these titles, please telephone 0870 787 1732 quoting reference 263H.
For further information about all Collins books, visit our website:
www.collins.co.uk**